RECOVERING A DIGITAL ADDICT

Your Guide to Beating Digital Addiction, Cyber Bullying, and More

Understand, Self-test and Take Action to Beat Digital Addiction, Cyber Bullying, Compulsive Behavior, Self-Comparison and more.

A comprehensive guide to understanding and addressing digital addiction, cyberbullying, compulsive behaviors, and the pitfalls of self-comparison in our hyper-connected world. Not only will you learn how to navigate these challenges personally, but also acquire the tools to assist others - your friends, children, students - in their own digital journeys. This handbook empowers you to be a beacon of knowledge and support, guiding those around you towards a balanced, healthy relationship with technology. Equip yourself and others with practical strategies, self-assessment tools, and actionable steps to turn the tide on harmful digital habits. Begin your collective journey towards a resilient, mindful digital life today.

A guide with strategies, self-tests, and a dedicated special section for parents.

BY S. B. SULZER

TABLE OF CONTENTS

We All Have a Role to Play

This book is about taking responsibility and giving back.

Media with adequate reach is power. I came to understand this at the age of 19 when my first article was published in a national newspaper. I was not happy with my article, but my editor told me, 'It is going to be read by millions, so it must be great if we publish it.' At that point, I started to feel the excitement of the potentially endless opportunities for growth and influence. Then reality hit. A few years later, when I became a leader of digital editorial teams across multiple countries, I realized what we were doing to people. We were working to glue them to screens, and our goal was to make them stay as long as possible. We utilized every opportunity, employed all the power and tools of social media and our platform, crafted the most engaging news and formats, and even developed new content types to reach our goal. Our efforts resulted in an enormous increase in the time spent in front of the screen by our readers. We delivered, but at what cost? I realized how unprepared the world was, and how unexpected the long-term impact of the growing power of media could be. The realization of what we as publishers, platforms, and influencers are actually doing to people was overwhelming. I quit.

Whether we're talking about the number of followers on social media, the viewers of a video, or the subscribers to a blog, what we're really discussing is the significant influence that these figures represent. In essence, each follower, viewer, or subscriber can be seen as a person who is potentially influenced by the content we share. Individuals in our society absorb, believe, and even shape their worldview based on the content they consume. It's a phrase we've all heard echoed, "I read it in the news," or "I saw it on Instagram," or "I found it on TikTok."

We must acknowledge and confront this reality: reach (the number of people we engage with our content on our platform in a given timeframe), the frequency of consumption, and time spent equate to power. With that power comes a significant responsibility. It is of utmost importance to be accountable for the content we disseminate, the messages we share with the world. It's equally essential to ensure outlets are held accountable for spreading misinformation or distributing content that can incite harm. The effects of such content can range from fostering false beliefs to provoking severe mental health issues, like depression or self-isolation. In the most alarming cases, it can even lead to catastrophic outcomes: suicides, mass shootings, or even precipitating wars. These are not hypothetical scenarios—they're real-world implications of the content that we, as media professionals, disseminate.

The technological revolution, an era of incredible progress and possibility, has also unleashed a beast. This beast was always present, lurking in the shadows, but our digital age has enabled it to emerge with frightening ease. Manipulating individuals of any age, fostering addictive behaviors, and compelling both adults and children to consume an increasing amount of content has become simpler than ever. This insatiable consumption can lead to a multitude of personal tragedies and widespread societal harm.

Just consider the impact of violent games on kids, or the barrage of celebrity news and trends that hit teenagers hard, leading them to compare themselves to 'trendy' celebrities and potentially develop body image disorders - these are just a few examples. Then, consider Elon Musk's influence on cryptocurrency. Merely by tweeting his support for certain currencies, he prompts people to invest and potentially suffer losses. There's also Vladimir Putin and his devastating war against Ukraine, launched based on false statements. And let's not forget Donald Trump's highly controversial use of social media. His tweets often stirred up division and spread misinformation, which eventually led to his ban from various platforms. Fox News also distributed disputed information about the 2020 US presidential election results, influencing millions of people, endangering US democracy, and thus interfering with the lives of every individual in the US. These are just a handful of examples. From Cambridge Analytica's data misuse to the proliferation of harmful content on platforms like TikTok, Facebook, and YouTube, numerous instances across the globe demonstrate the profound and often destructive influence of digital media. Where is the accountability for these actions, or for the effects they have caused?

Technology and the advent of the digital age have led to a drastic acceleration in the rate and volume of our content consumption. It's not just the content itself that can be harmful, but also the sheer volume of what we consume and the extensive amount of time we spend online. This can have detrimental effects on us and those around us. Therefore, using technology responsibly and being mindful of our digital balance are crucial steps we must take. However, the first step towards finding a solution is understanding and acknowledging these issues.

Science and technology are my passions, and to show that technology can be responsibly utilized for the greater good, I used the help of AI to write this book. My aim is to raise awareness, support people in their struggles, and provide possible solutions to help make a change. I wrote this book because I believe it's time for a change. As someone who has been part of this system, I feel a deep-seated responsibility to shed light on the issues we're facing.

Through this book, we will explore these issues in depth, striving to comprehend the full extent of Digital Addiction and its impact on our society. We will dive into our collective responsibility as media professionals and consumers, highlighting the necessity for change and the path we must take to ensure a healthier digital future. Our goal is not just to understand the problem but to illuminate the possibilities for action. Because the power of media should serve us, not exploit us. This responsibility is ours to shoulder. This change is ours to drive.

My hope is that this book will serve as a catalyst for a change, igniting conversations, inspiring action, and encouraging us to reclaim control of our digital lives. We all have a role to play in this journey, and it starts with acknowledging the power and responsibility that comes with our engagement in the digital world. Together, we can navigate this 'Digital Pandemic', and in doing so, build a digital future that is inclusive, ethical, and truly beneficial for us all.

How Did We End Up Here

The Digital Age

The Digital Age, also known as the Information Age or the New Media Age, is a period marked by the rapid evolution of technology, the growth of the internet, and the increasing role of digital devices in our lives. This era has brought about significant changes in the way we communicate, work, learn, and entertain ourselves. While it has undeniably introduced numerous benefits, it has also led to various challenges that affect our mental health and well-being. In this brief overview, we will explore the key developments that have shaped the Digital Age and discuss their implications for our lives.

The Rise of Personal Computers and the Internet

One of the most significant milestones in the Digital Age was the invention of the personal computer (PC) in the 1970s, which made computing accessible to a broader audience. The development of graphical user interfaces and the increasing affordability of PCs in the 1980s and 1990s further fueled their widespread adoption. This period also saw the birth of the World Wide Web, which transformed the internet from a tool used primarily by researchers and academics to a global phenomenon that revolutionized communication, commerce, and information sharing.

The proliferation of the internet led to the emergence of new communication channels, such as email and instant messaging, which allowed people to connect with one another regardless of their physical location. Online forums, chat rooms, and social networking sites also provided platforms for us to share ideas, opinions, and experiences, creating new opportunities for collaboration and community-building.

The Mobile Revolution

The turn of the 21st century witnessed another technological breakthrough that would change the face of the Digital Age: the advent of the smartphone. Combining the capabilities of a computer, a phone, and a camera, smartphones brought unprecedented convenience and accessibility to our lives. With the development of mobile applications and the growth of mobile internet, smartphones quickly became an indispensable tool for communication, information consumption, entertainment, and productivity.

As smartphone ownership soared, the mobile revolution also gave rise to new digital platforms and services, such as social media, streaming services, and e-commerce. These platforms have not only transformed our daily habits but have also spawned entirely new industries and business models. From ride-hailing services like Uber to short-term accommodation platforms like Airbnb, the digital economy has disrupted traditional industries and reshaped our expectations of convenience and connectivity.

The Era of Big Data and Artificial Intelligence

The Digital Age has generated an enormous amount of data, as our online activities leave behind a digital footprint that can be analyzed and used for various purposes. The rise of big data and advanced analytics has enabled companies to gain insights into consumer behavior, optimize their operations, and develop new products and services tailored to individual preferences. This data-driven approach has also paved the way for the development of artificial intelligence (AI) and machine learning, which have the potential to revolutionize industries ranging from healthcare and finance to transportation and manufacturing.

While AI has the potential to improve our lives in countless ways, it also raises concerns about privacy, security, and the ethical implications of using algorithms to make decisions that affect people's lives. As AI and machine learning continue to advance, it is crucial to strike a balance between leveraging their benefits and addressing the challenges they pose.

The Impact of the Digital Age on Society

The Digital Age has profoundly affected nearly every aspect of our lives, from the way we communicate and work to how we consume information and entertainment. While it has undeniably brought about numerous benefits, it has also introduced challenges that need to be addressed. On the one hand, it has provided us with unprecedented access to knowledge, opportunities for collaboration, and the ability to stay connected with friends and family across the globe. On the other hand, it has raised concerns about issues such as information overload, digital addiction, privacy, and the erosion of interpersonal skills.

Unprecedented Access to Information and Global Connectivity

One of the most significant advantages of the Digital Age is the unprecedented access to information and knowledge. The internet has made it possible for people to learn almost anything, from formal education through online courses to informal learning via blogs, podcasts, and videos. This democratization of knowledge has created new opportunities for personal and professional growth, allowing us to acquire new skills, explore different interests, and even change careers.

Global connectivity has also facilitated collaboration, enabling people from diverse backgrounds and geographical locations to work together on projects, share ideas, and form new communities. Social media platforms, in particular, have played a crucial role in connecting people and fostering a sense of belonging, both in personal relationships and professional networks.

Challenges and Concerns

Despite its many advantages, the Digital Age has also given rise to various challenges and concerns. One such issue is information overload, which occurs when people are exposed to more information than they can effectively process. This constant bombardment of information can lead to stress, anxiety, and decision fatigue, as we struggle to keep up with the latest news, trends, and updates.

Another concern is the growing prevalence of digital addiction and compulsive behaviors associated with technology use. People can become overly reliant on their devices, leading to negative consequences for their mental health, relationships, and overall well-being. Excessive screen time and social media use, for instance, have been linked to feelings of isolation, depression, and anxiety.

Privacy and security are also major concerns in the Digital Age, as the vast amount of personal data being shared and stored online raises questions about data protection and surveillance. The increasing sophistication of cyber threats, such as hacking, identity theft, and online harassment, further underscores the importance of developing robust digital privacy and security measures.

Furthermore, the Digital Age has raised concerns about the potential erosion of interpersonal skills and empathy, as face-to-face interactions are increasingly replaced by digital communication. This shift can lead to misunderstandings, misinterpretations, and a lack of emotional connection, which can negatively impact relationships and social cohesion.

Navigating the Digital Age

As we continue to navigate the complexities of the Digital Age, it is essential to strike a balance between embracing the benefits of technology and addressing the challenges it poses. This includes developing strategies for managing information overload, fostering digital well-being, and promoting healthy technology use. It also involves cultivating digital literacy and critical thinking skills, which can help us navigate the vast array of information available online and make informed decisions about our digital lives.

Moreover, it is crucial to prioritize privacy and security, both at the individual and societal levels, to ensure that the digital world remains a safe and empowering space. Finally, it is essential to foster empathy and emotional intelligence in our digital interactions, as well as promote the value of face-to-face communication and authentic human connections.

The Digital Age has brought about significant changes in the way we live, work, and interact with one another. While it has undeniably introduced numerous benefits, it has also presented challenges that need to be addressed. By adopting a balanced approach, we can harness the potential of technology to enhance our lives while mitigating its potential negative effects on our mental health and well-being.

The Double-Edged Sword of Technology

Technology has undoubtedly transformed our lives in myriad ways, bringing about significant advancements and conveniences that have changed the way we live, work, and communicate. However, this rapid evolution also presents challenges and concerns, particularly when it comes to mental health and well-being. We will delve into the positive and negative aspects of technology and explore the complex relationship between our digital lives and our mental health.

The Positive Aspects of Technology

Access to information and education: One of the most significant benefits of technology is the democratization of information and knowledge. The internet has made it possible for us to access vast amounts of information, which can be used for personal growth, education, and skill development. Online courses, tutorials, and educational resources have made learning more accessible and affordable than ever before, breaking down barriers and opening up new opportunities.

Global communication and connectivity: Technology has revolutionized communication, allowing people to connect instantly with friends, family, and colleagues around the world. Social media platforms, video conferencing, and messaging apps have made it easier than ever to maintain relationships, collaborate on projects, and share experiences, fostering a sense of global community and interconnectedness.

Enhanced productivity and efficiency: Digital tools and applications have significantly improved productivity and efficiency across various industries and personal endeavors. From project management software to automation and AI-driven solutions, technology has streamlined processes, reduced human error, and enabled us and organizations to achieve more with less effort.

Increased access to healthcare and mental health support: Technology has also played a pivotal role in improving access to healthcare and mental health support. Telemedicine, online therapy, and mental health apps have made it easier for us to seek professional help and access resources for managing our well-being, regardless of geographical location or financial constraints.

The Negative Aspects of Technology

Information overload and decision fatigue: The constant bombardment of information and stimuli in the Digital Age can lead to information overload, as we struggle to process and filter the vast amounts of data they encounter daily. This overload can contribute to stress, anxiety, and decision fatigue, negatively impacting mental health and well-being.

Screen time and physical health: Excessive screen time has been linked to various health issues, including sedentary lifestyles, obesity, and sleep disturbances. Studies have shown that prolonged exposure to screens, particularly before bedtime, can disrupt sleep patterns and negatively impact mental health.

Social comparison and self-esteem: Social media platforms, while fostering connectivity, can also contribute to feelings of inadequacy, envy, and low self-esteem, as we are constantly exposed to curated and filtered versions of others' lives. This social comparison can exacerbate mental health issues such as anxiety, depression, and body image concerns.

Digital addiction and compulsive behavior: The ubiquitous nature of digital devices and the design of many online platforms can lead to addictive behaviors and compulsive usage. Excessive engagement with technology, such as gaming, social media, or smartphone use, can have detrimental effects on mental health, relationships, and overall well-being.

Cyberbullying and online harassment: The anonymity and ease of communication afforded by the internet have given rise to new forms of bullying and harassment. Cyberbullying can have severe and long-lasting effects on the mental health of victims, leading to anxiety, depression, and even suicidal ideation.

Privacy concerns and mental health implications: The erosion of privacy in the Digital Age can contribute to feelings of vulnerability and anxiety, as we worry about our personal information being compromised or misused. This heightened sense of vulnerability can exacerbate existing mental health issues and contribute to new ones.

Technology is indeed a double-edged sword, offering numerous benefits while also presenting challenges to mental health and well-being.

The Importance of Digital Well-being

In today's fast-paced and interconnected world, digital devices have become an integral part of our daily lives. From smartphones and laptops to tablets and wearables, technology has transformed the way we communicate, work, learn, and consume information. While the benefits of technology are undeniable, the increasing reliance on digital devices also raises concerns about their impact on our mental health and well-being. We will explore the concept of digital well-being and discuss why it is crucial to address the effects of technology on our mental health.

Digital Well-being

Digital well-being refers to the optimal state of mental and emotional health that arises from the mindful and balanced use of digital devices and technology. It encompasses various aspects, including:

1. Managing screen time and setting boundaries for technology use
2. Cultivating healthy online habits and relationships
3. Protecting one's privacy and security
4. Developing digital literacy and critical thinking skills
5. Engaging in activities that promote mental and emotional well-being, both online and offline
6. The Relevance of Digital Well-being in the Modern World

Given the increasing prevalence of digital devices in our daily lives, it is crucial to address the impact of technology on mental health and well-being for several reasons:

The pervasiveness of technology: As digital devices become more and more ingrained in our lives, it becomes increasingly important to ensure that our interactions with technology are healthy and sustainable. From work and education to socializing and leisure activities, technology touches nearly every aspect of our lives, making it essential to prioritize digital well-being to maintain a sense of balance and mental health.

The influence of technology on mental health: Numerous studies have shown that excessive use of digital devices and specific online behaviors can contribute to mental health issues such as anxiety, depression, and sleep disturbances. By focusing on digital well-being, we can mitigate the negative effects of technology on our mental health and promote healthier digital habits.

The impact of technology on relationships: Digital devices and platforms have transformed the way we interact with one another, both positively and negatively. While technology has made it easier to stay connected with friends and family, it can also lead to feelings of isolation, loneliness, and a decline in face-to-face communication skills. Prioritizing digital well-being can help foster more authentic and meaningful connections with others, both online and offline.

The role of technology in self-esteem and self-perception: Social media platforms, in particular, have been linked to issues related to self-esteem, body image, and self-perception, as users are exposed to curated and filtered images of other people's lives. By focusing on digital well-being, we can develop a more realistic and healthy relationship with technology and social media, promoting a positive sense of self-worth and self-image.

The need for privacy and security in the digital age: With the increasing amount of personal information shared and stored online, privacy and security concerns have become a critical aspect of digital well-being. Protecting one's privacy and ensuring the security of personal data can help alleviate feelings of vulnerability and anxiety associated with the digital world.

Strategies for Promoting Digital Well-being

To address the impact of technology on mental health and well-being, we can adopt various strategies and practices that promote digital well-being:

Establish boundaries for technology use: Setting limits on screen time, creating device-free zones, and scheduling regular breaks from technology can help maintain a healthy balance between digital and offline activities.

Engage in digital detoxes: Periodically disconnecting from digital devices and participating in activities that promote mindfulness, relaxation, and mental rejuvenation can help counteract the negative effects of technology on mental health.

Cultivate healthy online habits: Developing a mindful approach to online behavior, such as setting specific goals for technology usage and engaging in positive digital interactions, can help foster a more balanced and beneficial digital experience. By consciously managing our digital habits, we can mitigate the negative effects of technology on our mental health and well-being, and ultimately create a more positive online environment.

Practice mindful social media use: Being intentional about the time spent on social media platforms, curating one's feed to include positive and inspiring content, and limiting engagement with content that triggers negative emotions can help foster a healthier relationship with social media.

Prioritize face-to-face interactions: Making an effort to engage in face-to-face communication and nurturing offline relationships can help counteract the potential negative effects of digital communication on interpersonal skills and emotional well-being.

Develop digital literacy and critical thinking skills: Being able to effectively evaluate the credibility of online sources, recognize misleading information, and navigate the vast array of digital content can help us make informed decisions about our digital lives and protect our mental health.

Implement privacy and security measures: Taking steps to protect personal information online, such as using strong passwords, enabling two-factor authentication, and being cautious about sharing sensitive information, can contribute to a sense of digital well-being and alleviate anxiety related to privacy concerns.

Seek professional help when necessary: If technology use is negatively impacting mental health and well-being, it may be helpful to consult a mental health professional or counselor who can provide guidance and support in developing healthier digital habits.

Encourage open dialogue about digital well-being: Discussing the impact of technology on mental health and well-being with friends, family, and colleagues can help raise awareness and foster a collective understanding of the importance of digital well-being.

Promote digital well-being in the workplace and educational settings: Employers and educators can play a crucial role in promoting digital well-being by implementing policies and initiatives that encourage a healthy balance between work and personal life, as well as providing resources and support for employees and students who may be struggling with the impact of technology on their mental health.

Given the increasing prevalence of digital devices in our daily lives, it is essential to address the impact of technology on mental health and well-being. By adopting strategies that promote digital well-being, we can maintain a healthier balance between our online and offline lives, protect their mental health, and foster a more positive and fulfilling relationship with technology. As we continue to navigate the complexities of the digital age, prioritizing digital well-being will become increasingly important in ensuring that we can harness the benefits of technology while mitigating its potential negative effects on our mental health and well-being.

The Book's Objectives

As we dive into the exploration of the impact of technology on mental health and well-being, it is crucial to establish a clear understanding of the objectives of this book and define the audience.

This book is for everyone.

Raise awareness of the effects of technology on mental health and well-being: The primary objective of this book is to raise awareness of the impact that technology, particularly digital devices and online platforms, can have on our mental health and overall well-being. By providing a comprehensive overview of the positive and negative aspects of technology use, we aim to shed light on the importance of addressing the issue and adopting practices that promote digital well-being.

Provide practical strategies and recommendations for promoting digital well-being: This book will offer actionable advice and strategies that readers can implement in their daily lives to improve their digital well-being. These recommendations will be based on scientific research, expert opinions, and real-life experiences, ensuring that the guidance provided is grounded in evidence and practicality.

Encourage open dialogue and reflection on personal technology use: Through the exploration of various topics related to digital well-being, this book aims to encourage readers to reflect on their own technology use and consider the ways in which it may be impacting their mental health and overall well-being. By fostering self-awareness and critical thinking, we hope to empower ourselves to take control of our digital lives and make informed decisions about our technology habits.

Support mental health professionals, educators, and parents in addressing digital well-being: The book also aims to serve as a valuable resource for mental health professionals, educators, and parents who are seeking to better understand the impact of technology on mental health and well-being. The strategies and recommendations provided will offer guidance on how to address digital well-being in various settings, such as therapy, the classroom, or at home.

Dear Reader,

This book is for you if you seek to improve your digital well-being. For those who are experiencing the negative effects of technology on their mental health and well-being, or are simply interested in cultivating healthier digital habits, will find this book particularly useful. The practical strategies and recommendations provided will offer guidance on how to achieve a more balanced and fulfilling digital life.

Educators: Teachers, school counselors, and administrators who are concerned about the impact of technology on their students' mental health and well-being will benefit from the insights and recommendations provided in this book. The content will offer guidance on how to address digital well-being in the classroom and support students in navigating the challenges of the digital age.

Parents: As technology becomes increasingly pervasive in the lives of children and adolescents, parents play a crucial role in fostering digital well-being within their families. This book will provide parents with the knowledge and tools they need to support their children in developing healthy digital habits and mitigating the negative effects of technology on their mental health.

By cultivating a deeper comprehension of the intricate interplay between technology and mental health, I aim to motivate readers to implement changes in both their personal and professional lives. This will encourage digital well-being and help establish a healthier, more balanced relationship with technology for themselves and those they interact with. In essence, this book functions as a crucial guide for navigating the trials and triumphs of the digital era, enabling readers to leverage the advantages of technology while minimizing its potential adverse impacts on mental health and well-being.

The Psychology of Screen Time

The Impact on Attention, Focus, and Information Overload

As our lives become increasingly intertwined with technology, the amount of time we spend interacting with screens has grown dramatically. While these devices offer numerous benefits and have revolutionized the way we communicate, work, and access information, their impact on our cognitive abilities, particularly attention and focus, cannot be overlooked.

The Effects of Screen Time on Attention and Focus

Distractions and Multitasking: With the constant barrage of notifications, emails, and messages vying for our attention, digital devices often create an environment ripe for distractions. The need to multitask between various tasks or applications can fragment our focus, making it difficult to concentrate on a single task for extended periods. Research has shown that multitasking can impair our cognitive abilities, resulting in reduced productivity and increased mental fatigue.

Decreased Attention Span: As we become more reliant on technology, our attention spans appear to be shrinking. With a wealth of information at our fingertips, we may be more prone to skim through content rather than engage deeply with it. This shift in information consumption can have negative consequences for our ability to process and retain information, ultimately impacting our attention spans and cognitive functioning.

Digital Dependency: The ease and convenience of digital devices can foster a sense of dependency, where we find ourselves constantly checking our phones, emails, or social media feeds. This digital dependency can make it challenging to detach from screens and focus on other tasks or activities, ultimately impacting our attention and focus.

Information Overload and Cognitive Strain

The Burden of Excessive Information: The proliferation of digital devices and the internet has led to an exponential increase in the amount of information available to us. This constant influx of data can create a sense of information overload, where our brains struggle to process, organize, and retain the vast amounts of incoming information.

Impaired Decision-Making and Critical Thinking: Information overload can lead to cognitive strain, which may impair our decision-making and critical thinking abilities. As we are bombarded with more information than we can effectively process, we may resort to cognitive shortcuts or rely on heuristics to make decisions, potentially leading to suboptimal choices or increased susceptibility to cognitive biases.

Increased Stress and Mental Fatigue: The constant pressure to stay informed and connected can contribute to increased stress and mental fatigue. Information overload, coupled with the demands of multitasking and the need to maintain constant attention, can leave us feeling overwhelmed and mentally exhausted.

The impact of screen time on our attention, focus, and ability to manage information overload is a critical issue that warrants attention and consideration. By understanding these effects and the potential consequences on our cognitive functioning, we can make more informed decisions about our digital habits and implement strategies to mitigate the negative effects of screen time.

Sleep and Circadian Rhythms

Sleep is a vital component of our overall health and well-being, playing a crucial role in maintaining our physical, emotional, and cognitive functioning. As screen time continues to dominate our daily lives, it's essential to understand how our interaction with digital devices can impact our sleep patterns and circadian rhythms.

The Effects of Screen Time on Sleep Patterns

Blue Light Exposure: Digital devices, such as smartphones, tablets, and computers, emit a type of high-energy visible (HEV) blue light that has been found to disrupt our natural sleep-wake cycle. Exposure to blue light during the evening hours can suppress the production of melatonin, the hormone responsible for regulating sleep, making it more difficult to fall asleep and stay asleep throughout the night.

Nighttime Device Usage: Engaging with screens close to bedtime can negatively impact our sleep quality and duration. Activities such as watching videos, browsing social media, or playing games can stimulate our minds and make it harder to unwind and fall asleep. Additionally, the constant barrage of notifications and alerts can create a sense of urgency and anxiety, further disrupting our ability to relax and prepare for sleep.

Sleep Disruption and Sleep Disorders: Excessive screen time, particularly before bedtime, has been linked to various sleep disruptions and sleep disorders, such as insomnia and sleep apnea. Poor sleep quality can have significant repercussions on our overall health and well-being, including impaired cognitive functioning, mood disturbances, and weakened immune systems.

The Impact on Circadian Rhythms

Circadian Rhythm Disruption: Our circadian rhythms, also known as our internal body clocks, regulate various physiological processes, including our sleep-wake cycle. Exposure to blue light from digital devices, particularly in the evening, can disrupt our natural circadian rhythms, leading to difficulties falling asleep, frequent nighttime awakenings, and daytime sleepiness.

The Importance of Maintaining a Consistent Sleep Schedule: Consistently using digital devices late into the night can cause irregular sleep patterns, making it challenging to maintain a consistent sleep schedule. A stable sleep schedule is essential for optimal health, as it ensures that our body's internal processes are synchronized and functioning effectively.

The influence of screen time on sleep patterns and circadian rhythms is a critical concern that requires careful consideration. By understanding the impact of blue light exposure and nighttime device usage, we can make more informed choices about our digital habits and prioritize the importance of quality sleep. Implementing practical strategies, such as establishing a consistent bedtime routine, reducing screen time before bed, and using blue light-filtering applications or devices, can help mitigate the adverse effects of screen time on sleep and circadian rhythms.

Social Comparison, Online Validation, and Mental Health

The rise of social media and the ubiquity of digital devices have transformed the way we interact with others and perceive ourselves. With access to a constant stream of updates, images, and information about the lives of others, the tendency to engage in social comparison and seek online validation has become increasingly prevalent. We will investigate the psychological effects of social comparison, online validation, and the relationship between excessive screen time and mental health issues.

Social Comparison and Its Impact

The Nature of Social Comparison: Social comparison is a natural human tendency to evaluate ourselves in relation to others, often to determine our standing or worth within a particular domain. While social comparison can sometimes serve as a source of motivation or inspiration, it can also lead to negative emotions, such as envy, dissatisfaction, and low self-esteem.

The Role of Social Media: Social media platforms are fertile grounds for social comparison, as they provide users with curated highlights of others' lives, often presenting an unrealistic and idealized representation of reality. These carefully crafted images can create a distorted sense of what is normal or attainable, leading users to compare themselves to unrealistic standards and feel inadequate or discontented.

Emotional Consequences: Engaging in social comparison on social media can have significant emotional consequences. Studies have shown that frequent social comparison, particularly through social media platforms, can lead to increased feelings of envy, depression, and loneliness, as well as a decrease in overall life satisfaction.

Online Validation and Its Effects

The Pursuit of "Likes" and Approval: As social media has become increasingly intertwined with our daily lives, the pursuit of online validation, often in the form of "likes," comments, and shares, has gained importance for many of us. This quest for validation can lead to an overemphasis on external approval and an unhealthy reliance on the opinions of others to determine self-worth.

The Impact on Self-Esteem: The constant quest for online validation can have a significant impact on an individual's self-esteem. When we base our self-worth on the feedback and approval of others, our self-esteem can become fragile and susceptible to fluctuations based on external factors. This can lead to feelings of insecurity, self-doubt, and a diminished sense of self-worth.

Fear of Missing Out (FOMO): The desire for online validation can also contribute to the phenomenon known as the Fear of Missing Out (FOMO). FOMO is the uneasy feeling that others are experiencing more fulfilling lives or having more fun than you are, often fueled by the curated content displayed on social media. This fear can lead to increased anxiety, feelings of inadequacy, and a compulsion to stay constantly connected.

The Relationship Between Screen Time and Mental Health

The Connection to Anxiety and Depression: Research has shown that excessive screen time, particularly on social media platforms, is associated with increased levels of anxiety and depression. This connection can be attributed to various factors, including the negative emotional consequences of social comparison, the pursuit of online validation, and the impact of screen time on sleep and circadian rhythms.

The Link to Addiction: The constant need for connection and online validation can foster addictive behaviors, we become reliant on digital devices and social media platforms to fulfill our emotional needs. This digital addiction can have a detrimental impact on mental health, personal relationships, and overall well-being.

The psychological effects of social comparison, online validation, and excessive screen time on mental health are multifaceted and warrant close attention. By understanding these dynamics and their potential consequences, we can make more informed choices about our digital habits and develop strategies for promoting a healthier, more balanced relationship with technology.

Strategies for Mindful Screen Use and Digital Detox

As we become more aware of the potential adverse effects of excessive screen time on our mental health and well-being, it's essential to develop strategies to manage our digital habits and foster a healthier relationship with technology. See some practical tips and recommendations for effectively managing screen time, incorporating digital detoxes, and promoting mindful screen use.

Setting Boundaries and Limitations

One of the most effective ways to manage screen time is to set clear boundaries and limitations on when and how we engage with digital devices. Consider the following approaches:

1. Designate specific times for screen use: Establish dedicated periods for engaging with digital devices, such as during designated breaks or specific hours in the evening. By setting aside specific times for screen use, we can create a more structured and mindful approach to technology.

2. Implement device-free zones: Designate certain areas in your home or workplace as device-free zones, such as the bedroom, dining room, or any space where you wish to encourage focused, present-moment activities.

3. Use technology to manage technology: Utilize built-in screen time management tools or third-party applications to monitor and limit your screen time. These tools can help you gain insight into your digital habits and set limits on specific apps or activities.

Prioritize Mindful Screen Use

To foster a healthier relationship with technology, it's essential to prioritize mindful screen use. This involves engaging with digital devices intentionally and purposefully, rather than mindlessly scrolling or multitasking. Consider the following strategies:

1. Be intentional with your screen time: Before engaging with a digital device, take a moment to ask yourself why you are picking it up and what you hope to accomplish. By setting a clear intention for your screen use, you can help ensure that your time spent on screens is purposeful and meaningful.

2. Focus on one task at a time: Avoid multitasking while using digital devices, as this can contribute to fragmented attention and cognitive overload. Instead, focus on one task or activity at a time, allowing yourself to fully engage with the content and minimize distractions.

3. Practice active consumption: When engaging with digital content, aim to be an active rather than passive consumer. This might involve taking notes, engaging in thoughtful discussions, or reflecting on the information presented.

Incorporating Digital Detoxes

Periodically taking a break from digital devices, also known as a digital detox, can be an effective way to reset and regain balance in our relationship with technology. Consider the following approaches for incorporating digital detoxes into your routine:

1. Schedule regular digital detoxes: Plan regular intervals for digital detoxes, such as one day per week, one weekend per month, or even a full week each year. By incorporating these breaks into your schedule, you can create a consistent and sustainable approach to managing screen time.

2. Engage in alternative activities: During your digital detox, make an effort to engage in activities that do not involve screens, such as reading physical books, spending time in nature, or participating in hobbies and creative pursuits.

3. Involve friends and family: Encourage your friends and family to join you in your digital detox efforts, as this can provide a supportive environment and help hold you accountable. Additionally, engaging in shared experiences without screens can help strengthen personal relationships and create lasting memories.

Promoting Digital Well-being

In addition to managing screen time and incorporating digital detoxes, it's essential to prioritize digital well-being by fostering a healthy and balanced relationship with technology. Consider the following tips:

1. Focus on quality over quantity: When engaging with digital content, prioritize quality over quantity. Seek out content that is informative, inspiring, or beneficial to your personal growth, rather than mindlessly consuming content that provides little value.

2. Use technology for personal growth: Leverage technology to support your personal and professional development. This might involve using online resources for learning new skills, connecting with like-minded individuals, or accessing tools that promote productivity and organization.

3. Be mindful of social media usage: Pay attention to the impact that social media has on your mental health and well-being. Consider unfollowing or muting accounts that trigger negative emotions, focusing on content that uplifts and inspires you, and limiting the time you spend on social media platforms.

4. Foster genuine connections: While technology can facilitate communication and connection, it's essential to prioritize genuine, face-to-face interactions with others. Make an effort to engage in meaningful conversations and activities with friends, family, and colleagues without the interference of screens and digital devices.

Cultivating a Balanced Relationship with Technology

Ultimately, managing screen time and promoting digital well-being involves cultivating a balanced and healthy relationship with technology. This may require a combination of the strategies discussed above, as well as a commitment to ongoing self-reflection and adjustment as needed. Consider the following practices to support your journey towards digital well-being:

1. Regularly assess your digital habits: Periodically evaluate your digital habits, paying attention to any patterns or behaviors that may be negatively impacting your mental health and well-being. This might involve tracking your screen time, journaling about your experiences, or reflecting on your emotional state during and after engaging with digital devices.

2. Set personal goals: Establish personal goals related to screen time and digital well-being, and monitor your progress towards achieving these goals. These might include reducing your overall screen time, incorporating more device-free activities into your routine, or engaging with technology more mindfully and intentionally.

3. Remain open to change: As you work towards cultivating a balanced relationship with technology, remain open to change and willing to adapt your strategies as needed. This might involve trying new techniques, seeking support from others, or reassessing your goals and priorities as your relationship with technology evolves.

Effectively managing screen time, incorporating digital detoxes, and fostering a healthier relationship with technology is essential for promoting mental health and well-being in today's digital age. By implementing the strategies discussed, you can take control of your digital habits, prioritize digital well-being, and create a more balanced and fulfilling life. As you continue on this journey, remember that cultivating a healthy relationship with technology is an ongoing process that requires self-awareness, commitment, and persistence.

The Dark Side of Constant Connectivity

Always-On Culture: The Societal Expectations of Constant Connectivity

In today's fast-paced world, constant connectivity has become the norm. The proliferation of smartphones, tablets, and other digital devices has made it easy for people to stay connected around the clock. However, the societal expectations that come with this always-on culture have led to a range of negative consequences for mental health and well-being. Let's into the issues arising from constant connectivity, including overwork, burnout, and the subsequent effects on mental health.

The Pressure to Be Always Connected

The widespread adoption of digital devices has enabled people to stay connected with friends, family, and colleagues at any time and from any location. However, this constant connectivity comes with a price. Many of us feel a growing pressure to be available 24/7, whether it's for work or social reasons. This pressure to be constantly connected can lead to a feeling of being "on" all the time, with little opportunity for rest or downtime.

Overwork and Burnout

As a result of the always-on culture, many of us find ourselves working longer hours and experiencing heightened stress levels.The boundaries between work and personal life often blur, making it difficult to switch off and relax, even when not working. This relentless pace can contribute to overwork and eventually lead to burnout, a state of emotional, physical, and mental exhaustion caused by prolonged and excessive stress.

Burnout not only affects job performance but also has significant implications for mental health. Symptoms of burnout may include feelings of cynicism, detachment, and a sense of ineffectiveness. In more severe cases, burnout can lead to anxiety, depression, and other mental health disorders.

Sleep Disruption and Digital Devices

The constant connectivity enabled by digital devices also has a significant impact on sleep patterns and overall sleep quality. Many people find it difficult to resist the urge to check their devices right before bed or even in the middle of the night. The use of screens close to bedtime can disrupt the body's natural circadian rhythms, making it more challenging to fall asleep and stay asleep.

Moreover, the blue light emitted by digital screens has been shown to suppress melatonin production, a hormone that helps regulate sleep. Consequently, those who frequently use digital devices before bedtime may experience increased stress, fatigue, and anxiety due to poor sleep quality and insufficient rest.

The Connection Between Screen Time and Stress

Research has demonstrated a link between excessive screen time and heightened stress and anxiety levels. Spending long hours in front of screens can contribute to feelings of overwhelm and information overload. Constant exposure to the internet and social media can also create unrealistic expectations and promote social comparison, leading to increased stress and anxiety.

In the long term, excessive screen time and the resulting stress can have serious implications for mental health. Studies have found that people with high screen time are at a greater risk of developing mental health disorders such as anxiety and depression.

Strategies for Managing Constant Connectivity

To counter the negative effects of constant connectivity on mental health and well-being, it is essential to develop strategies for effectively managing one's relationship with digital devices. Some practical tips and recommendations include:

1. Set boundaries: Establish clear boundaries between work and personal life. Set specific times for checking emails and social media, and avoid using devices during designated rest periods.

2. Prioritize sleep: Prioritize sleep by creating a bedtime routine that promotes relaxation and minimizes screen time. Avoid using digital devices at least an hour before bedtime to allow the body and mind to wind down.

3. Practice mindfulness: Engage in mindfulness practices such as meditation or yoga to help manage stress and anxiety. Mindfulness can help us become more aware of our thoughts and feelings, enabling us to respond to stressors more effectively.

4. Take regular breaks: Schedule regular breaks throughout the day to step away from screens and digital devices. Use this time to engage in activities that promote relaxation and well-being, such as going for a walk, practicing deep breathing exercises, or simply enjoying a cup of tea.

5. Create a technology-free zone: Designate a specific area in your home or workspace as a technology-free zone. This can be a space where you can relax and recharge without the distractions of digital devices.

5. Engage in digital detoxes: Consider taking regular digital detoxes, during which you disconnect from digital devices for a set period of time. This can be as short as a few hours or as long as several days, depending on your needs and preferences. Digital detoxes can help you regain control over your relationship with technology and create a healthier balance in your life.

6. Cultivate offline hobbies and interests: Develop hobbies and interests that do not involve digital devices, such as reading, painting, or playing a musical instrument. Engaging in activities that do not require screens can help reduce stress and promote overall well-being.

8. Foster genuine connections: While digital devices can help us stay connected with others, it is essential to prioritize in-person interactions and foster genuine connections. Spending quality time with friends and family without the interference of screens can help strengthen relationships and promote emotional well-being.

The dark side of constant connectivity is an important topic to address, as the consequences for mental health and well-being can be severe. By understanding the negative impacts of the always-on culture and adopting strategies to manage constant connectivity, we can foster a healthier relationship with technology and improve our overall mental health and well-being.

Sleep Disruption and Digital Devices

The widespread use of digital devices has revolutionized the way we live, work, and communicate. However, this constant connection to screens has also led to significant disruptions in sleep patterns, ultimately affecting our quality of rest and well-being.

The Role of Digital Devices in Sleep Disruption

There are several ways in which digital devices can disrupt sleep patterns and negatively impact the quality of rest. Some of the key factors include:

Blue light exposure: Digital devices, such as smartphones, tablets, and laptops, emit a blue light that has been shown to suppress melatonin production, the hormone responsible for regulating sleep. Exposure to blue light in the evening can interfere with the body's natural circadian rhythms, making it more difficult to fall asleep and stay asleep.

Mental stimulation: Engaging with digital devices before bed can lead to mental stimulation, which may make it challenging to relax and wind down before sleep. Activities such as checking emails, scrolling through social media, or playing games can keep the mind active, making it harder to transition into a restful state.

Sleep environment: The use of digital devices in the bedroom can disrupt the sleep environment, creating a space that is not conducive to rest. The presence of screens and the constant influx of notifications can make it difficult to establish a peaceful and calming atmosphere, which is essential for a good night's sleep.

The Consequences of Sleep Disruption

Sleep disruption caused by digital devices can lead to a variety of negative consequences for mental health and well-being, including:

Increased stress: Poor sleep quality can contribute to heightened stress levels, as the body is unable to effectively recover and recharge during the night. This can lead to a vicious cycle, as increased stress can further disrupt sleep patterns, exacerbating the problem.

Fatigue: Insufficient rest can result in feelings of fatigue and exhaustion, affecting daily functioning and productivity. Persistent fatigue can impair decision-making abilities and increase the risk of accidents and errors.

Anxiety: Sleep disruptions have been linked to increased anxiety levels, as the body's natural stress response is activated when it is unable to achieve sufficient rest. Over time, chronic sleep disruptions can contribute to the development of anxiety disorders.

Impaired cognitive function: Sleep is essential for maintaining optimal cognitive function, including memory, learning, and attention. Disrupted sleep patterns can negatively impact these cognitive processes, leading to difficulties with focus, problem-solving, and retaining new information.

Sleep Disruption Self-Test

Constant connectivity to digital devices can have a significant impact on our sleep patterns. The light emitted by screens, the mental stimulation from content, and the habit of using devices before bedtime can all contribute to sleep disruption. This self-test will help you assess whether your digital device usage might be affecting your sleep quality.

Sleep Disruption Self-Test Scoring System

For each of the following statements, score yourself as follows:

- 0 points: I have never experienced this.
- 1 point: I have rarely experienced this.
- 2 points: I occasionally experience this.
- 3 points: I frequently experience this.

Score the following statements:

1. I use digital devices within an hour of going to bed.
2. I find it difficult to fall asleep after using digital devices.
3. I wake up during the night to check my phone or other digital devices.
4. I feel the urge to respond to notifications, messages, or emails just before going to sleep.
5. I have trouble staying asleep throughout the night after using digital devices.
6. I feel tired, groggy, or unrested upon waking up in the morning.
7. I feel the need to use digital devices as a way to relax or unwind before sleep.
8. My mind feels active or overstimulated after using digital devices at night.
9. I spend more time on digital devices than I initially intended, cutting into my sleep time.
10. I have difficulty concentrating or staying alert during the day due to poor sleep.

Scoring

- 0-5 points: Low level of sleep disruption. Your digital device usage seems to have minimal impact on your sleep quality. Continue to practice good sleep hygiene and be mindful of your device usage before bedtime.
- 6-15 points: Moderate level of sleep disruption. Some aspects of your digital device usage may be affecting your sleep quality. Consider implementing strategies to reduce screen time before bed, such as setting limits or creating a device-free bedtime routine.
- 16-30 points: High level of sleep disruption. It is likely that your digital device usage is significantly impacting your sleep quality. It's important to take action to improve your sleep hygiene, such as creating a consistent sleep schedule, establishing a relaxing bedtime routine without devices, and turning off notifications at night. If your sleep issues persist, consider speaking with a healthcare professional for further guidance.

Strategies to Mitigate Sleep Disruption from Digital Devices

To reduce the impact of digital devices on sleep patterns and overall well-being, several strategies can be implemented:

1. Establish a screen-free bedtime routine: Create a consistent bedtime routine that does not involve digital devices. This can include activities such as reading a physical book, taking a warm bath, or practicing relaxation techniques, such as deep breathing or meditation.

2. Limit blue light exposure: Reduce exposure to blue light in the evening by using blue light filters on digital devices or wearing blue light-blocking glasses.

3. Set a digital curfew: Establish a specific time in the evening to stop using digital devices, allowing for an adequate wind-down period before sleep.

4. Keep devices out of the bedroom: Remove digital devices from the bedroom to create a more calming and restful sleep environment. Consider using a traditional alarm clock instead of a smartphone to wake up in the morning.

The impact of digital devices on sleep patterns and quality of rest is a growing concern in today's constantly connected world. By understanding the ways in which screens can disrupt sleep and implementing strategies to mitigate these effects, we can promote healthy sleep habits and improve overall mental health and well-being. As we continue to navigate the digital age, it is essential to strike a balance between our reliance on technology and the need for quality rest. By prioritizing sleep and implementing practical steps to minimize the negative effects of digital devices, we can foster a healthier relationship with technology and enjoy the benefits it provides while preserving our physical and emotional well-being.

The Connection Between Screen Time and Stress

In today's digital age, screen time has become an integral part of our daily lives. The ubiquity of smartphones, tablets, and computers allows for constant connectivity, enabling us to work, communicate, and access information at all times. However, this constant engagement with digital devices has also been linked to increased stress and anxiety levels. See the connection between excessive screen time and heightened stress, the potential long-term impacts on mental health, and strategies for managing screen time to mitigate these effects.

The Link Between Screen Time and Stress

Research has shown a correlation between excessive screen time and increased stress levels. Some of the primary factors contributing to this relationship include:

Information overload: The constant barrage of information from emails, social media, and news sources can lead to cognitive overload, making it difficult to process and retain information effectively. This can cause feelings of overwhelm, frustration, and anxiety.

Multitasking: The use of digital devices often encourages multitasking, as we switch between apps, respond to messages, and engage with various types of media simultaneously. Multitasking has been shown to increase stress levels and reduce productivity, as it is more difficult to focus and complete tasks efficiently.

Fear of missing out (FOMO): The prevalence of social media and the constant stream of updates from friends, family, and influencers can lead to a fear of missing out on events, experiences, or opportunities. This can cause feelings of inadequacy and anxiety, driving us to spend more time on digital devices to stay connected and up to date.

Work-related stress: The ability to access work-related content and communicate with colleagues outside of regular working hours can blur the lines between work and personal life, leading to increased stress and a reduced ability to disconnect and relax.

Long-term Impacts on Mental Health

The connection between screen time and stress is not only relevant for immediate well-being but also has potential long-term implications for mental health. Some of these long-term impacts include:

Chronic stress: Prolonged exposure to stressors, such as excessive screen time, can lead to chronic stress, which has been linked to a range of mental health issues, including depression, anxiety disorders, and sleep disturbances.

Impaired cognitive function: As mentioned earlier, excessive screen time can lead to cognitive overload, reducing the brain's ability to process and retain information effectively. Over time, this can result in impaired cognitive function, which may contribute to the development of mental health issues.

Social isolation: Increased screen time can contribute to social isolation, as we may spend less time engaging in face-to-face interactions and more time connecting through digital devices. Social isolation has been linked to a variety of mental health issues, including depression and anxiety.

Addictive behaviors: Excessive screen time has been associated with the development of addictive behaviors, such as compulsive smartphone use or internet addiction. These addictive behaviors can have negative consequences for mental health, leading to increased stress, anxiety, and depression.

Strategies for Managing Screen Time and Reducing Stress

To mitigate the impact of screen time on stress levels and mental health, several strategies can be implemented:

Set limits on screen time: Establish boundaries around screen time, such as setting specific times of day for using digital devices, avoiding screens during meals or before bedtime, and scheduling regular breaks throughout the day.

Prioritize face-to-face interactions: Encourage meaningful social connections by engaging in face-to-face interactions with friends, family, and colleagues. This can help to counteract the potential negative effects of social isolation and promote emotional well-being.

Practice mindfulness: Incorporate mindfulness practices, such as meditation or deep breathing exercises, to help manage stress and reduce the impact of screen time on mental health. Mindfulness can help us become more aware of their thoughts and emotions, allowing us to better manage stressors and cultivate a healthier relationship with technology.

Create a screen-free environment: Designate specific areas of the home or workspace as screen-free zones, where digital devices are not allowed. This can help to promote relaxation and create a more balanced environment for mental well-being.

Engage in physical activity: Regular exercise has been shown to reduce stress and anxiety levels while improving overall mental health. Incorporating physical activity into your daily routine can help counteract the negative effects of excessive screen time.

Develop healthy sleep habits: Prioritize quality sleep by establishing a consistent sleep schedule, creating a relaxing bedtime routine, and avoiding screen time before bed. This can help to improve sleep quality and reduce the impact of digital devices on stress and mental health.

Seek professional help: If screen time-related stress is causing significant distress or impacting daily functioning, it may be beneficial to consult with a mental health professional, such as a therapist or counselor, for support and guidance.

The connection between excessive screen time and heightened stress levels is an important consideration for us as we navigate the digital age. By understanding the potential long-term impacts on mental health and implementing strategies to manage screen time effectively, we can foster a healthier relationship with technology and promote overall well-being. It is essential to strike a balance between the convenience and benefits provided by digital devices and the need to protect and prioritize our mental health.

Strategies for Managing Constant Connectivity

In today's fast-paced world, the ability to disconnect from digital devices and manage constant connectivity has become increasingly important for maintaining mental health and well-being. A healthy relationship with technology is essential to avoid the negative consequences of constant connectivity, such as stress, anxiety, and burnout.

Set boundaries around technology use

Establishing clear boundaries around technology use is crucial for maintaining a healthy balance between the digital world and the real world. Some suggestions for setting boundaries include:

1. Designate specific times for checking emails, social media, and other digital platforms. By limiting the frequency of these interactions, you can reduce the urge to constantly check your devices and create more focused, intentional periods of connectivity.

2. Turn off non-essential notifications on your devices. By reducing the number of distractions and interruptions throughout the day, you can create a more focused and peaceful environment.

3. Establish screen-free zones in your home or workspace, where digital devices are not allowed. This can help to create a more balanced environment for relaxation and productivity.

Prioritize face-to-face interactions

In an age of constant connectivity, it is essential to prioritize face-to-face interactions and maintain strong interpersonal connections. Some ways to prioritize in-person interactions include:

1. Schedule regular social activities and outings with friends and family, making an effort to keep digital devices out of sight during these gatherings.

2. Make an effort to have meaningful conversations with coworkers or classmates, rather than relying solely on digital communication.

3. Engage in community events or join local clubs and organizations to connect with others and foster a sense of belonging.

Practice digital detoxes

Regularly disconnecting from digital devices, or participating in a "digital detox," can help to reset your relationship with technology and promote a healthier balance between online and offline activities. Some ideas for digital detoxes include:

1. Set aside specific days or weekends where you commit to staying off your devices.

2. Participate in activities that do not involve technology, such as hiking, reading, or engaging in hobbies.

3. If a full digital detox feels too challenging, try gradually reducing screen time or implementing device-free periods throughout the day.

Incorporate mindfulness and self-care

Practicing mindfulness and self-care can help to manage the stress and anxiety associated with constant connectivity. Some suggestions for incorporating mindfulness and self-care into your daily routine include:

1. Engage in regular meditation or deep breathing exercises to help cultivate awareness and manage stress.

2. Practice gratitude by reflecting on the positive aspects of your life, rather than focusing solely on the digital world.

3. Prioritize self-care activities such as exercise, proper nutrition, and adequate sleep, which can help to alleviate stress and improve overall well-being.

Cultivate a growth mindset

Developing a growth mindset, or the belief that abilities and intelligence can be developed through dedication and hard work, can help to create a more balanced relationship with technology. By focusing on personal growth and development, you can build resilience and better cope with the challenges associated with constant connectivity. Some ways to cultivate a growth mindset include:

1. Embrace challenges and view them as opportunities for growth and learning, rather than as insurmountable obstacles.

2. Practice self-compassion and self-acceptance, recognizing that setbacks are a natural part of the learning process.

3. Seek out opportunities for personal and professional development, such as attending workshops, conferences, or taking online courses.

Managing constant connectivity is essential for maintaining mental health and well-being in the digital age. By implementing practical strategies such as setting boundaries, prioritizing face-to-face interactions, engaging in digital detoxes, and practicing mindfulness and self-care, you can foster a healthier relationship with technology and mitigate the potential negative effects of constant connectivity. Cultivating a growth mindset and focusing on personal development can further enhance your resilience and well-being in the face of technological challenges.

Ultimately, the key to managing constant connectivity lies in finding a balance that works for your individual needs and lifestyle. It is important to regularly evaluate your relationship with technology and make adjustments as needed to ensure that your digital habits are supporting, rather than hindering, your overall well-being.

By proactively addressing the challenges of constant connectivity, you can harness the many benefits of the digital age while maintaining a strong sense of mental health and well-being. In doing so, you will be better equipped to navigate the complex landscape of the digital world, cultivating a more balanced, healthy, and fulfilling life both online and offline.

Social Media and Mental Health

Social Media and Self-Esteem

In the digital age, social media platforms have become an integral part of our daily lives. While these platforms offer numerous benefits, such as connecting with friends and family, sharing our experiences, and gaining access to information, they can also have a significant impact on our self-esteem. Explore the ways in which social media can affect our self-esteem, focusing on the quest for validation, the presentation of an idealized self, and the comparison trap.

The Quest for Validation: Likes, Comments, and Shares

Social media platforms are designed to encourage engagement through features such as likes, comments, and shares. These features can provide a sense of validation and social approval, making us feel connected and valued by our peers. However, this quest for validation can also have negative consequences for our self-esteem, as we may begin to rely on external validation to define our self-worth.

The dopamine effect: Receiving likes, comments, and shares can trigger the release of dopamine, a neurotransmitter associated with pleasure and reward. This can lead to an addictive cycle, where we constantly seek out more validation to maintain this pleasurable feeling.

The impact on self-worth: Over time, our self-esteem may become increasingly dependent on the validation we receive from others through social media. This can lead to feelings of insecurity and a diminished sense of self-worth when we do not receive the expected level of engagement on our posts.

Strategies for overcoming the quest for validation: To break the cycle of seeking validation through social media, it's essential to develop a healthy sense of self-worth that is not dependent on external approval. This can involve practicing self-compassion, focusing on personal growth, and engaging in activities that build self-esteem outside of the digital realm.

The Curated Self: Presenting an Idealized Version Online

Social media allows us to present a carefully curated version of ourselves to the world, selecting the aspects of our lives we wish to highlight and share. This can lead to the creation of an idealized self-image, which may not accurately reflect our true selves.

The pressure to be perfect: The desire to present an idealized version of ourselves can create pressure to maintain a perfect image on social media. This can lead to feelings of inadequacy and low self-esteem when we compare our real lives to the curated lives of others.

The impact on authenticity: The constant pressure to maintain an idealized self-image can also impact our authenticity, as we may feel compelled to hide or downplay our flaws, challenges, and struggles.

Strategies for embracing authenticity: To foster a healthier relationship with social media and our self-esteem, it's essential to embrace authenticity and vulnerability. This can involve sharing our struggles and challenges alongside our achievements, practicing self-acceptance, and focusing on meaningful connections with others.

The Comparison Trap: The Impact of Constant Comparison on Self-Esteem

Social media can fuel our natural tendency to compare ourselves to others, leading to a perpetual cycle of comparison that can negatively impact our self-esteem.

Upward and downward comparison: social media exposes us to both upward comparisons (comparing ourselves to those who appear to be more successful, attractive, or happy) and downward comparisons (comparing ourselves to those who appear to be less fortunate). While downward comparisons can temporarily boost our self-esteem, upward comparisons often lead to feelings of inadequacy and diminished self-worth.

The impact on self-esteem: Constantly comparing ourselves to others on social media can contribute to feelings of envy, dissatisfaction, and low self-esteem. This can be particularly damaging when we compare our real lives to the curated, idealized lives of others.

Strategies for overcoming the comparison trap: To break free from the cycle of constant comparison on social media, consider implementing the following strategies:

1. Limit exposure: Be intentional about the time you spend on social media, setting boundaries and scheduling specific times to engage with these platforms. This can help to reduce the frequency of comparisons and their impact on your self-esteem.

2. Focus on personal growth: Shift your focus from comparing yourself to others to concentrating on your own personal growth and development. Engage in activities that promote self-improvement and self-compassion, such as journaling, meditation, or pursuing new hobbies and interests.

3. Cultivate gratitude: Practice gratitude by regularly reflecting on the positive aspects of your life, as well as the unique qualities and experiences that make you who you are. This can help to counteract the negative effects of comparison and foster a greater appreciation for your own life and accomplishments.

4. Seek meaningful connections: Focus on building and maintaining genuine connections with others, both online and offline. Engage in conversations that go beyond superficial topics and foster a sense of community and mutual support.

Social media can have a significant impact on our self-esteem, particularly through the quest for validation, the presentation of an idealized self, and the comparison trap. By recognizing these potential pitfalls and implementing strategies to address them, we can cultivate a healthier relationship with social media and foster greater self-esteem in our daily lives. Ultimately, it's essential to remember that our self-worth should not be defined by the validation we receive from others, but rather by our own personal growth, achievements, and authentic connections with others.

Social Comparison and Social Media

Social comparison is a fundamental aspect of human psychology, as we constantly evaluate ourselves in relation to others. While social comparison can sometimes serve as a motivational force for self-improvement, it can also have negative effects on our well-being when it becomes excessive or unhealthy. We will now explore the nature of social comparison, how social media fuels this tendency, and strategies for managing social comparison on social media platforms.

The Nature of Social Comparison: Upward and Downward Comparisons

Social comparison can be divided into two main categories: upward and downward comparisons. Understanding the differences between these types of comparisons can help us to better navigate our online interactions and manage their impact on our well-being.

Upward comparisons: Upward comparisons occur when we compare ourselves to those who appear to be more successful, attractive, or happy than ourselves. These comparisons can lead to feelings of envy, inadequacy, and low self-esteem.

Downward comparisons: In contrast, downward comparisons involve comparing ourselves to those who appear to be less fortunate, less successful, or facing greater challenges. While these comparisons can sometimes provide a temporary boost to our self-esteem, they can also foster negative emotions such as guilt, pity, or complacency.

Social Media as a Breeding Ground for Comparison

Social media platforms provide ample opportunities for social comparison, as we are constantly exposed to the curated lives of others. The unique features of social media can amplify the effects of social comparison, leading to increased feelings of inadequacy and dissatisfaction.

Selective self-presentation: Social media encourages users to present their best selves, often leading to the curation of idealized images and experiences. This can create an environment where we are constantly comparing ourselves to the seemingly perfect lives of others, exacerbating feelings of inadequacy and low self-esteem.

The impact of algorithms: Social media algorithms are designed to prioritize content that is likely to generate engagement, often leading to an overrepresentation of success stories, extraordinary experiences, and idealized images. This can create a distorted view of reality, fueling social comparison and its negative effects on our well-being.

Strategies for Managing Social Comparison on Social Media

To mitigate the negative effects of social comparison on social media, consider implementing the following strategies:

1. Awareness and self-reflection: Develop an awareness of your own tendencies to engage in social comparison, and reflect on how these comparisons make you feel. Recognize when you are comparing yourself to others and challenge the validity of these comparisons by reminding yourself that social media often presents a distorted view of reality.

2. Limit exposure: Set boundaries around your social media use, such as scheduling specific times for engagement or reducing the number of platforms you use. This can help to limit the opportunities for social comparison and its impact on your well-being.

3. Curate your feed: Be intentional about the content and accounts you follow, prioritizing those that inspire, uplift, and promote a healthy and realistic view of life. This can help to create a more balanced and positive social media experience, reducing the negative effects of comparison.

4. Practice self-compassion: Cultivate a compassionate attitude towards yourself, recognizing that everyone has strengths and weaknesses, successes and failures. Remind yourself that your self-worth is not determined by your social media presence or how you compare to others, but rather by your own personal growth, values, and authentic connections.

Social comparison is a natural human tendency, but it can have negative consequences when it becomes excessive or unhealthy, particularly on social media platforms. By understanding the nature of social comparison, recognizing the ways in which social media fuels this tendency, and implementing strategies to manage social comparison, we can foster a healthier relationship with social media and promote greater well-being in our digital lives.

It's essential to recognize that the curated lives we see on social media are not an accurate reflection of reality, and that comparing ourselves to these idealized images can lead to feelings of inadequacy, envy, and low self-esteem. Instead, we should strive to focus on our own personal growth, accomplishments, and authentic connections with others.

By cultivating self-awareness, self-compassion, and mindfulness in our social media use, we can mitigate the negative effects of social comparison and create a more balanced, positive, and empowering online experience. Ultimately, our goal should be to use social media as a tool for connection, inspiration, and personal growth, rather than allowing it to dictate our self-worth and well-being.

Fear of Missing Out (FOMO) and Social Media

Fear of Missing Out (FOMO) is a pervasive psychological phenomenon that has become particularly prevalent in the digital age. It refers to the anxiety or discomfort experienced when we believe that others may be having rewarding experiences that we are not a part of. Social media has significantly contributed to the amplification of FOMO, as it provides a constant stream of information about the lives and activities of others. See the psychology of FOMO, the role of social media in exacerbating it, and tips for overcoming FOMO in the digital age.

The Psychology of FOMO: Causes and Consequences

Causes: FOMO often arises from a combination of factors, including the desire for social connection, the need for social validation, and the inherent human tendency to compare ourselves to others. These factors are exacerbated by the constant exposure to the curated lives of others through social media platforms.

Consequences: FOMO can have a range of negative consequences on our mental health and well-being, including increased feelings of loneliness, anxiety, and dissatisfaction with our lives. It can also lead to compulsive social media use, as we constantly seek reassurance that we are not missing out on important experiences or events.

The Role of Social Media in Exacerbating FOMO

Instant access to information: Social media platforms provide instant access to the lives and activities of others, making it easy for us to constantly compare ourselves and feel as though we are missing out on exciting experiences or events.

The curated nature of social media content: Social media encourages users to share only the highlights of their lives, creating an idealized version of reality that can foster feelings of inadequacy and FOMO.

The fear of social exclusion: Social media can amplify the fear of social exclusion, as we are constantly reminded of the social events and gatherings we are not a part of, leading to increased feelings of FOMO and anxiety.

Strategies for Overcoming FOMO in the Digital Age

1. Limit social media exposure: Set boundaries around your social media use, such as scheduling specific times for engagement or reducing the number of platforms you use. This can help to limit the opportunities for FOMO to develop and reduce its impact on your well-being.

2. Practice mindfulness: Engage in mindfulness practices, such as meditation or deep breathing exercises, to help you stay present and focused on your own experiences, rather than constantly seeking validation and reassurance through social media.

3. Cultivate gratitude: Develop a daily gratitude practice, reflecting on the positive aspects of your life and the experiences you have had. This can help to counteract the negative effects of FOMO and foster a greater appreciation for your own life.

4. Focus on authentic connections: Rather than obsessing over the lives of others, invest your time and energy in cultivating genuine connections with friends and loved ones, both online and offline. This can help to alleviate feelings of FOMO and promote a greater sense of belonging and social connection.

FOMO is a common psychological phenomenon that has been exacerbated by the rise of social media. By understanding the underlying causes and consequences of FOMO, and implementing strategies to manage it, we can create a healthier relationship with social media and foster greater well-being in our digital lives. Ultimately, the key is to focus on cultivating authentic connections, engaging in mindfulness practices, and appreciating the experiences and relationships that enrich our lives, rather than constantly comparing ourselves to others and feeling as though we are missing out.

FOMO, Self-Esteem, and Social Comparison Self-Test

Social media can have profound effects on our mental health. While it offers opportunities for connection and communication, it can also foster a sense of FOMO, impact self-esteem, and provoke harmful social comparisons. This self-test will help you gauge the potential impact of your social media use on these aspects of your mental well-being.

Self-Test Scoring System

For each of the following statements, score yourself as follows:

- 0 points: This never applies to me.
- 1 point: This rarely applies to me.
- 2 points: This sometimes applies to me.
- 3 points: This often applies to me.
- 4 points: This always applies to me.

Statements

1. I feel anxious if I can't check my social media regularly.

2. I find myself comparing my life to the lives of others I see on social media.

3. I feel left out or excluded when I see posts of events I did not attend.

4. I feel bad about myself when I see others' achievements or success on social media.

5. I feel that my life is not as good as others' due to what I see on social media.

6. I spend more time on social media than I feel is healthy for me.

7. I have difficulty disconnecting from social media, even when it's time for bed or work.

8. I feel a need to share or post frequently to feel connected and valued.

9. I base my self-worth on the number of likes, comments, or shares I get.

10. I fear missing out on news, events, or popular trends if I don't check my social media.

Scoring

- 0-10 points: Low impact. Your social media use seems to have minimal negative effects on your FOMO, self-esteem, and tendency for social comparison. Continue practicing mindful social media use.

- 11-25 points: Moderate impact. Some aspects of your social media use may be affecting your FOMO levels, self-esteem, and tendency for social comparison. It might be helpful to set boundaries for social media use and engage in activities that bolster your self-esteem off-line.

- 26-40 points: High impact. Your social media usage appears to be significantly impacting your FOMO levels, self-esteem, and prompting social comparison. Consider seeking guidance on how to navigate your social media use in a healthier manner. This may involve creating a healthier social media environment, setting usage boundaries, or seeking professional help if necessary.

Building Resilience and Promoting Mental Health on Social Media

The pervasive influence of social media on our lives can have both positive and negative effects on our mental health and well-being. It is crucial to develop resilience and adopt strategies that promote mental health while engaging with social media platforms. We will explore the process of developing a healthy social media mindset, setting boundaries and limiting exposure, and fostering genuine connections while focusing on personal growth.

Developing a Healthy Social Media Mindset

Be mindful of comparison: Remind yourself that social media platforms often showcase only the highlights of others' lives, and comparing yourself to these idealized portrayals can lead to feelings of inadequacy and unhappiness.

Cultivate self-awareness and self-compassion: Practice self-awareness and self-compassion when engaging with social media, acknowledging your feelings and emotions without judgment and treating yourself kindly.

Focus on your values and priorities: Align your social media use with your personal values and priorities, ensuring that the time you spend online is genuinely contributing to your personal growth and well-being.

Setting Boundaries and Limiting Exposure

Schedule specific times for social media use: Designate specific times during the day for engaging with social media, and avoid mindlessly scrolling during moments of boredom or downtime.

Limit the number of platforms: Reduce the number of social media platforms you actively engage with, focusing on those that genuinely add value to your life and align with your interests and values.

Implement digital detoxes: Regularly engage in digital detoxes, taking breaks from social media and digital devices to recharge and reconnect with your offline life.

Fostering Genuine Connections and Focusing on Personal Growth

Engage in meaningful interactions: Prioritize engaging in meaningful interactions with friends and loved ones on social media, rather than seeking validation through likes, comments, and shares.

Share authentically: Be mindful of the content you share on social media, ensuring that it reflects your true self and promotes genuine connections with others.

Invest in personal growth: Use social media as a tool for personal growth and development by following accounts that inspire and educate, rather than provoke feelings of inadequacy or envy.

Building resilience and promoting mental health on social media requires a combination of strategies, including developing a healthy mindset, setting boundaries, and fostering genuine connections. By implementing these practices, we can create a more balanced, positive, and empowering online experience that supports our overall well-being. Ultimately, the key is to engage with social media in a mindful, intentional manner, focusing on personal growth and authentic connections rather than allowing it to dictate our self-worth and happiness.

Digital Addiction and Compulsive Behavior

Understanding Digital Addiction and Compulsive Behavior

Digital addiction and compulsive behavior have been hot topics in the realm of psychology and behavioral health over the past decade. As we become more entwined with technology in our daily lives, understanding the psychological implications of this relationship becomes increasingly important. In this discussion, we'll define these concepts, explore the psychology behind them, consider their most common manifestations, and address the scale of the problem.

Digital addiction, also known as Internet or tech addiction, is characterized by an individual's inability to regulate their use of digital devices, to the point where it significantly interferes with life activities. Compulsive behavior, on the other hand, is an irresistible urge to behave in a certain way, often against one's conscious wishes. In the context of digital addiction, compulsive behavior often manifests as repeated and excessive use of digital devices or platforms.

The psychology behind digital addiction and compulsive behavior is complex and multifaceted. At its core, it often involves a process known as operant conditioning. The brain's reward system is triggered by certain activities, such as receiving likes or comments on social media or achieving high scores in a video game. This results in the release of dopamine, a neurotransmitter associated with feelings of pleasure and satisfaction. Over time, the brain may start to crave these digital interactions, and we may find it difficult to resist the urge to engage in these behaviors, even when they negatively impact other areas of life.

There are several common manifestations of digital addiction. These include excessive use of social media platforms, compulsive online gaming, and uncontrolled online shopping. Each of these behaviors has its unique characteristics, but they share common traits: they provide immediate gratification or reward, they can be accessed anytime and anywhere, and they can result in a significant amount of time being spent on these activities.

Social media addiction is often driven by the desire for social connection and validation, while gaming addiction may be fueled by the thrill of competition and achievement. Online shopping addiction, meanwhile, can stem from the pleasure of acquiring new items and the convenience of online retail.

The scale of the problem of digital addiction and compulsive behavior is substantial and growing. While exact prevalence rates can vary depending on the criteria used to define addiction, it's clear that a significant number of people struggle with managing their digital behavior. Research suggests that certain demographic groups, such as adolescents and young adults, may be particularly vulnerable due to their high levels of technology use and their ongoing cognitive and emotional development.

However, it's crucial to remember that digital addiction and compulsive behavior are not limited to these groups. As digital devices become ever more ingrained in our lives, all age groups are at risk. Thus, understanding and addressing digital addiction and compulsive behavior is a societal concern requiring collective effort.

Digital addiction and compulsive behavior are complex issues that are increasingly relevant in our digital age. By understanding the psychology behind these behaviors, their manifestations, and their prevalence, we can better equip ourselves to address these challenges and promote healthier relationships with technology.

The Role of Dopamine and the Reward System in Digital Addiction

The increasing prevalence of digital addiction has pushed researchers to explore the underlying biological mechanisms that contribute to this phenomenon. Central to this exploration is the role of dopamine, a neurotransmitter, and the brain's reward system. We will dive into how these biological elements contribute to digital addiction, the effects of intermittent reinforcement on compulsive behavior, and the similarities between digital addiction and other forms of addiction.

Dopamine is a neurotransmitter, a type of chemical messenger in the brain, that plays a crucial role in how we perceive pleasure and reward. It's released when we engage in activities that our brains perceive as beneficial or enjoyable, such as eating, exercising, or socializing. This dopamine release is the brain's way of teaching us to repeat these beneficial behaviors. However, dopamine also plays a central role in the development of addiction, including digital addiction.

In the context of digital addiction, activities such as scrolling through social media, receiving likes or comments, winning a level in an online game, or making an online purchase trigger the release of dopamine. This creates a sensation of pleasure and satisfaction, teaching our brains to repeat these activities to experience the pleasure again. Over time, the brain may begin to crave these digital interactions, creating a cycle of dependency akin to the processes observed in substance addiction.

Intermittent reinforcement, or the unpredictable or inconsistent delivery of rewards, is another factor that contributes to compulsive behavior in digital addiction. Many digital platforms are designed to provide rewards (such as likes, comments, or notifications) unpredictably, which can make the experience more exciting and addictive. This is similar to how a slot machine works, providing unpredictable rewards that keeps us engaged and repeatedly pulling the lever. This unpredictable reward system can intensify the addictive nature of digital platforms, making it harder for us to disengage.

The similarities between digital addiction and other forms of addiction, such as substance abuse or gambling addiction, are striking. All these forms of addiction involve a dysregulation of the brain's reward system and an over-reliance on certain behaviors or substances for dopamine release. Just as a person with a substance addiction may require increasing amounts of the substance to experience the same level of pleasure (a phenomenon known as tolerance), a person with a digital addiction may find themselves spending increasing amounts of time online to achieve the same level of satisfaction. Furthermore, just as people with substance addiction may experience withdrawal symptoms when they stop using the substance, people with digital addiction may experience restlessness, irritability, or discomfort when they try to reduce their screen time.

Understanding the role of dopamine and the brain's reward system in digital addiction provides valuable insights into the biological underpinnings of this phenomenon. This knowledge can help inform effective strategies for managing digital addiction, with an emphasis on promoting healthier dopamine release through beneficial activities and reducing dependence on digital platforms for gratification. Ultimately, fostering a balanced and mindful relationship with technology is crucial in the digital age.

Digital Addiction & Compulsive Behavior Self-Test

Having explored the intricate dynamics of dopamine and the reward system in the context of digital addiction, we now comprehend how our brains innately crave rewarding experiences. We've come to recognize how digital technologies can exploit these desires, furnishing us with incessant stimuli, immediate satisfaction, and unpredictable rewards. As we've seen, these biochemical reactions can progressively cultivate behavioral patterns akin to addiction over time.

While digital technology has undoubtedly brought about immense benefits, it's also important for us to remain aware of its potential pitfalls. One such pitfall is digital addiction, a term that refers to the compulsive use of digital devices to the point where it interferes with our lives. This can manifest in various ways, such as excessive screen time, the inability to cut down usage, or persistent technology-related behaviors despite experiencing negative consequences.

To gain a better understanding of our relationship with digital technology and evaluate if we may be at risk of digital addiction, we have developed a simple self-test. This self-test is designed to help us reflect on our digital habits and assess whether our use of digital devices might be moving into the territory of problematic behavior.

As you navigate through the questions, remember that honesty is key. This is not a diagnostic tool, but a starting point for introspection and self-awareness. If you find that your score indicates a high level of digital addiction, we strongly recommend seeking professional help to navigate this challenge.

Digital Addiction Self-Test:

Rate the following statements on a scale of 1 to 5, with 1 being "Strongly Disagree" and 5 being "Strongly Agree".

1. I feel restless or uncomfortable when I am unable to use digital devices.
2. I find myself spending more time on digital devices than I intend to.
3. My use of digital devices interferes with my work, studies, or other important activities.
4. I often lose track of time when using digital devices.
5. I have tried to cut down on the use of digital devices but have been unsuccessful.
6. I often use digital devices to escape from negative feelings or problems.
7. I neglect other activities or responsibilities because of my digital device use.
8. I feel a need to use digital devices for increasing amounts of time to achieve satisfaction.
9. I have lied to others about how much time I spend on digital devices.
10. My use of digital devices has negatively affected my relationships.

Scoring:

10-19: Low level of digital addiction - Your digital habits may not be problematic, but it's always good to stay mindful of your use.

20-29: Moderate level of digital addiction - You may be at risk of digital addiction. Consider implementing strategies for healthier digital habits.

30-50: High level of digital addiction - Your digital habits appear to be significantly impacting your life. It would be beneficial to seek professional help to navigate this challenge.

Remember, it's not about completely eliminating digital devices from our lives, but about finding a balance that supports our well-being.

Consequences of Digital Addiction and Compulsive Behavior

Digital addiction and compulsive behaviors have far-reaching consequences, affecting not only us but also our relationships, work, and overall quality of life. The impact of digital addiction spans various domains, including mental health, daily life, long-term physical and psychological well-being, and social and professional performance.

Mental health consequences of digital addiction are significant and multifaceted. Research suggests strong links between excessive digital use and mental health disorders such as anxiety and depression. For example, constant exposure to curated and often idealized online personas can lead to feelings of inadequacy and low self-esteem. Also, the instant gratification provided by digital platforms can lead to decreased patience and increased frustration in the real world, contributing to heightened anxiety levels. Compulsive behaviors, such as constant checking of social media or emails, can also exacerbate stress levels. Furthermore, excessive screen time often translates to reduced time for real-world social interactions, leading to feelings of social isolation.

Digital addiction can also disrupt our relationships and daily life. When we spend too much time on screens, we might start to overlook our personal relationships, as we could begin to place more importance on online interactions rather than face-to-face connections. This can strain relationships with friends, partners, and family members, leading to conflicts and feelings of loneliness. Moreover, compulsive use of digital devices can disrupt daily routines and responsibilities, such as work or school tasks, personal hygiene, and even basic activities such as eating and sleeping.

The long-term physical and psychological consequences of digital addiction are equally concerning. Prolonged sedentary behavior associated with excessive screen time can lead to physical health issues such as obesity, cardiovascular disease, and musculoskeletal problems. The blue light emitted by screens can disrupt sleep patterns, leading to poor quality sleep, which in turn can contribute to various health problems, including weakened immune system, cognitive impairments, and mental health disorders. Psychologically, long-term digital addiction can lead to chronic stress, mood disorders, and even changes in brain structure and function similar to those seen in substance addiction.

Digital addiction also has serious social and academic/professional implications. In the academic realm, students who are excessively engaged in digital activities often experience decreased academic performance due to reduced study time and increased distraction. Similarly, in the workplace, digital addiction can lead to decreased productivity, increased error rates, and strained professional relationships. On a societal level, the widespread prevalence of digital addiction can lead to increased health care costs and decreased societal productivity.

The consequences of digital addiction and compulsive behavior are far-reaching and deeply concerning. They underscore the urgent need for public health interventions aimed at promoting healthier digital habits. It's critical to recognize the signs of digital addiction and seek professional help when necessary. Furthermore, as a society, we must foster a culture that values balance and mindful digital use, providing individuals with the tools and knowledge they need to navigate the digital world without compromising their mental, physical, and social well-being.

Strategies for Overcoming Digital Addiction and Compulsive Behavior

Overcoming digital addiction and compulsive behavior often starts with recognition and acceptance. It requires admitting the problem exists and acknowledging its impact on various facets of life. Recognizing digital addiction involves self-reflection and awareness of one's behavior patterns. Signs may include excessive time spent online, compulsive checking of social media or emails, neglect of personal relationships or responsibilities, and feelings of restlessness or irritability when unable to access digital devices. From denial to acceptance, this initial step is crucial as it opens the pathway to seek help and initiate change.

Professional help

Therapies and interventions can provide us with the essential tools and strategies to manage compulsive behaviors and lessen the impact of addiction. Cognitive-behavioral therapy (CBT), for instance, is particularly beneficial in addressing digital addiction. CBT assists us in understanding the thoughts and feelings that sway our behaviors, and offers coping strategies for handling addictive actions. Therapists may also utilize mindfulness-based therapies, inviting us to be fully present in the moment, thereby reducing the compulsion to engage with digital devices. In severe cases, more structured interventions, like residential treatment programs specializing in digital addiction, may be necessary.

Developing healthy coping mechanisms and alternative activities

Instead of turning to digital devices during times of boredom or stress, we can learn to engage in other rewarding activities. This might include physical exercise, which not only serves as a distraction but also releases endorphins, thus improving mood and reducing stress. Hobbies such as reading, painting, or playing a musical instrument can also provide a sense of fulfillment and satisfaction that digital interactions often lack. Social activities, like spending time with friends and family or volunteering in the community, can enhance real-world social connections and reduce feelings of isolation.

Setting boundaries and implementing digital detox strategies

This might involve designated technology-free times or zones, such as during meals or in the bedroom, to minimize distractions and promote healthier habits. It's also beneficial to remove unnecessary apps or notifications that trigger compulsive checking. Regular digital detoxes, periods during which one intentionally avoids using digital devices, can also be beneficial. This not only provides a break from constant digital stimulation but also allows us to reflect on our digital habits and reset our relationship with technology.

Building resilience and promoting long-term recovery
Resilience, the capacity to recover quickly from difficulties, can be strengthened by enhancing emotional well-being, nurturing healthy relationships, and developing a positive self-concept. Mindfulness practices, physical activity, and balanced nutrition contribute to overall well-being, while support from family, friends, and therapy groups fosters a sense of connection and community. Building resilience also involves learning to handle stress and setbacks without resorting to compulsive behaviors. This might involve using relaxation techniques, developing problem-solving skills, or seeking support from a therapist or support group.

Managing screen time and fostering conscious use of technology
There are a variety of tools and apps available that can help us monitor and control our screen time. These tools can provide insights into which activities consume the most time and can help set limits on certain applications. Conscious use of technology involves being mindful about why and how we're using digital devices. It encourages intentional and purposeful use of technology, such as using social media to connect with friends or using a smartphone to organize schedules, rather than mindless scrolling or compulsive checking.

Support systems play a significant role in combating digital addiction
The support of family, friends, and communities cannot be underestimated. Loved ones can provide encouragement, help set boundaries, and offer understanding during challenging times. They can also help the individual engage in alternative activities and social interactions. Additionally, joining a support group or online community for digital addiction can provide a sense of camaraderie, shared experiences, and practical tips for managing addictive behaviors.

Education and awareness

By educating ourselves, especially our younger generations, about the potential risks and consequences of excessive technology use, we can encourage healthier digital habits from the outset. This education should also extend to parents, teachers, and other influencers who can model healthy technology use and support children in their digital habits. Awareness campaigns, school curriculums, and community programs can play a significant role in this education process.

Overcoming digital addiction and compulsive behavior requires a multifaceted approach. Building resilience, managing screen time, relying on support systems, and promoting education and awareness are all crucial strategies in this process. It's a challenging journey, but with the right tools and support, we can reclaim control over our digital habits, improve our well-being, and lead a balanced and fulfilling life in the digital age. Remember, it's not about demonizing technology, but about fostering a healthier relationship with it.

Also, it is not a straightforward process, but a combination of recognition, professional help, alternative activities, and boundary setting can significantly improve one's relationship with technology. It's important to remember that it's not about completely eliminating technology, but rather about establishing a healthier, more balanced relationship with it.

Gaming and Mental Health

Introduction to Gaming Culture

The digital age brought with it an entertainment revolution, reshaping how we play, connect, and even learn. At the heart of this transformation is the world of video games. As immersive as it is diverse, the gaming culture has evolved from simple pixelated games on arcade machines to a global phenomenon spanning age groups, nationalities, and interests. Today, understanding this culture is no longer an option but a necessity for parents and caregivers.

Video gaming has its roots in the mid-20th century, but it wasn't until the late '70s and early '80s that it began to capture the public's imagination. With the introduction of home consoles and the advent of iconic games like Pac-Man, Space Invaders, and Super Mario, gaming stepped out from the shadow of a niche hobby and into the mainstream.

Fast forward to today, and the landscape is drastically different. The gaming industry now rivals and even surpasses Hollywood in terms of revenue. According to a report by the Entertainment Software Association, in 2022, the video game industry was valued at over $159.3 billion, a leap from just $17.5 billion in 2000. This exponential growth demonstrates not just the financial might of gaming, but its increasing significance in our daily lives.

Gaming culture itself is as varied as the games that populate it. Role-playing games (RPGs), for instance, make up about 25% of the total game market, enticing players with intricate storylines and character development. On the other hand, action and strategy games each account for approximately 22%, offering adrenaline-pumping experiences or tactical challenges. Then there are sports and racing games, educational games, and an array of mobile games, each with their unique appeal.

What makes these games particularly appealing to kids and teenagers? For starters, games are inherently interactive. Unlike watching TV or a movie, players are active participants in their entertainment. They can explore vast virtual worlds, complete challenging tasks, and engage in social interactions, all within the safety of their homes.

Moreover, many games, especially multiplayer ones, come with a strong social component. Players can team up with friends or make new ones, compete against each other, and even form communities, providing a sense of belonging. For many young individuals, these games are more than just leisure; they offer a platform for self-expression and connection.

As parents and caregivers, understanding the gaming culture is critical. This goes beyond simply knowing which games are popular or how to operate a console. It's about comprehending the attractions and the challenges of this digital environment. It involves grasping the psychological impact of games, how they can influence behavior, and how they can be a double-edged sword, offering both benefits and potential harm.

In the next section, we dive deeper into this topic, exploring the psychology of gaming. From the addictive design elements that keep players hooked to the emotional reactions games can incite, we'll offer insights to equip you with a better understanding of this immersive digital landscape.

The Psychology of Gaming

With a firm grasp of gaming culture, it's time to navigate the complex terrain of gaming psychology. At the core of this domain lie the powerful mechanics and features that keep players engrossed. To comprehend the addictive nature of games, it's crucial to understand these elements, namely: reward systems, leveling structures, and social features.

The Lure of the Reward System

Reward systems are the heart of any game. They tap into our brain's natural desire for achievement and gratification, creating a cycle that keeps players coming back for more. This system can manifest in various forms: earning points, unlocking new levels, acquiring unique items, or even just witnessing the progression of a storyline.

Underlying this is a psychological principle known as operant conditioning, first proposed by B.F. Skinner. According to this theory, an individual's behavior can be shaped by its consequences. If a behavior is followed by a reward, that behavior is more likely to be repeated.

When applied to gaming, the theory takes a compelling form. Complete a level, defeat an enemy, solve a puzzle – you earn rewards. This immediate gratification triggers the release of dopamine, a neurotransmitter associated with pleasure, thus reinforcing the behavior. However, game designers don't just use rewards abundantly; they often employ a variable ratio schedule, which means rewards are given out at unpredictable intervals. This unpredictability tends to produce a high, steady rate of response from players, fueling their desire to continue playing.

Leveling Up: An Endless Pursuit

Another integral aspect of the gaming world is the concept of 'levels.' Levels serve multiple functions: they provide a tangible measure of progress, offer increasing challenges, and, importantly, deliver a consistent sense of achievement.

As players ascend levels, they encounter new challenges, environments, and enemies, which help maintain interest and curiosity. Overcoming these challenges and 'leveling up' serves as a significant accomplishment, further pushing players to strive for the next milestone. The sense of progression and the prospect of new rewards make this a highly effective tool in sustaining player engagement.

Social Connection: A Double-Edged Sword

Lastly, social features play a crucial role in the appeal and potential addictiveness of games, especially in the era of online multiplayer games. Features such as team play, in-game chat, and leaderboards contribute to a social environment that goes beyond the game itself.

These social connections can be incredibly enriching, fostering teamwork, camaraderie, and communication. For many, especially introverted or socially anxious individuals, online games offer a safe space for interaction. However, the flip side of this social element can contribute to excessive gaming. The fear of missing out on in-game events, letting down team members, or falling behind on leaderboards can compel players to devote more time and emotional investment into the game than they initially intended.

Understanding these elements – reward systems, levels, and social features – illuminates the mechanics that make games so engaging and potentially addictive. However, this knowledge is not a condemnation of gaming. Instead, it provides a foundation to approach gaming in a mindful, balanced manner, fostering healthy habits while acknowledging the potential risks.

In subsequent sections, we dive into the impact of excessive gaming on mental health, explore the controversial connection between gaming and violence, and equip parents and caregivers with strategies to manage and prevent gaming addiction.

Mental Health Impacts of Gaming

As we dive deeper into the intricate world of gaming, it is important to shed light on the potential mental health impacts of excessive gaming. The nuances of these impacts are complex, involving elements of isolation, loneliness, and potential effects of in-game violence, which have been the subjects of much research and debate.

The Social Paradox: Isolation and Loneliness

Gaming, particularly online gaming, is inherently a social activity, yet it can also be a source of isolation and loneliness. How can this paradox exist?

The answer lies in the nature of digital interaction. Many gamers, especially those who spend extended hours engrossed in the gaming world, may find themselves gradually substituting face-to-face social interactions with digital ones. While gaming can provide an avenue for social engagement, it is fundamentally different from real-world interactions. It may foster feelings of connection during gameplay but can leave individuals feeling isolated and disconnected from the physical world.

The impact can be especially significant for young gamers who spend critical developmental years behind screens. The American Academy of Pediatrics warns that children spending too much time on digital media can lack crucial social skills needed for real-life social interactions.

Furthermore, prolonged gaming can be associated with feelings of loneliness. While moderate gaming can provide a valuable social platform, over-reliance on gaming as a primary source of socializing can result in feelings of loneliness and dissatisfaction.

In-game Violence and Its Impact on Young Minds

The impact of in-game violence on young minds has been a contentious issue, sparking debate among parents, researchers, and policymakers alike. Some studies suggest a link between exposure to violent video games and increased aggression in children and teenagers. However, it's critical to understand that aggression does not equate to violent behavior, a distinction often blurred in public discourse.

A report by the American Psychological Association (APA) highlighted this concern, stating that research has demonstrated a consistent relation between violent video game use and increases in aggressive behavior, aggressive cognitions, and aggressive affect. However, it also emphasized the lack of research to link violent video game play with criminal violence or youth violence.

It's important to remember that video games are just one of many factors that can influence the behavior and mindset of young individuals. Other factors, such as home environment, social interactions, and personal predispositions, can play significant roles as well.

Addressing the Mental Health Impacts of Gaming

Recognizing the potential mental health impacts of gaming is not about demonizing the gaming culture. Rather, it underscores the need for awareness, balance, and mindful engagement with this popular pastime. Parents and caregivers need to be proactive in understanding these potential impacts and fostering a healthier relationship between children and their digital worlds.

As we continue this discussion in subsequent sections, we'll explore the connection between gaming and addiction, dive deeper into the controversy surrounding gaming and violence, and provide valuable strategies to prevent and manage potential issues stemming from gaming.

The Connection Between Gaming and Addiction

Gaming, when enjoyed in moderation, can offer a creative, exciting outlet and even foster a sense of community. However, when it becomes excessive, it can also develop into a severe addiction, which is increasingly recognized in the realm of mental health. It's essential to understand how gaming can parallel other forms of addiction to ensure the prevention or early intervention for those who may be at risk.

Gaming Addiction: A Real Concern

In 2018, the World Health Organization officially recognized "gaming disorder" as a mental health condition, marking a significant shift in acknowledging the serious implications of excessive gaming. The characteristics of gaming addiction are similar to substance use disorders or gambling disorder, in that it involves a pattern of persistent or recurrent gaming behavior, indicated by impaired control over gaming, increasing priority given to gaming, and continuation of gaming despite negative consequences.

Why Does Gaming Become Addictive?

Like any addiction, the roots of gaming addiction are multifaceted. It often starts innocuously, with gamers initially playing for fun, social connection, or escapism. However, certain psychological mechanisms inherent in game design can contribute to its addictive nature.

Firstly, many games employ a system of rewards and progress, which provides a constant stream of achievement. As the gamer progresses, they unlock new levels, abilities, or items, which offers a sense of accomplishment and progression. This reward system can trigger the release of dopamine, a brain chemical associated with pleasure and reward, making the game increasingly enticing and stimulating.

Secondly, online multiplayer games offer a social dimension. Players can connect with friends or even strangers worldwide, forming teams or communities, which can become an important part of their social identity and life.

Lastly, for some players, gaming offers a refuge from real-life issues or stressors, a concept known as 'escapism.' While escapism is not inherently harmful, when gaming becomes the primary coping mechanism, it can lead to neglect of real-world responsibilities and relationships, contributing to the cycle of addiction.

Gaming Addiction Self-Test

Understanding the signs of gaming addiction is crucial for early intervention. These may include:

- Preoccupation with gaming
- Withdrawal symptoms when gaming is taken away

- Tolerance, meaning that more time needs to be spent gaming
- Unsuccessful attempts to quit or reduce gaming
- Loss of interest in other hobbies and activities
- Continued excessive gaming despite awareness of psychosocial problems
- Deceiving family members or others regarding the amount of time spent on gaming
- Use of gaming to escape or relieve negative moods
- Jeopardizing or losing significant relationships, jobs, or educational opportunities due to gaming
- If you or someone you know is exhibiting these signs, it might be time to seek help.

Remember, the goal isn't to vilify games but to promote a balanced and mindful approach towards gaming.

Answer the following questions honestly, choosing the one that best describes your behavior in relation to gaming in the past 12 months. Each response has a score:

Never: 1 point
Rarely: 2 points
Sometimes: 3 points
Often: 4 points
Very Often: 5 points

1. Do you spend a lot of your free time thinking about games or planning how to play the next game?
2. Do you feel restless, irritable, moody, angry, anxious or sad when attempting to cut down or stop gaming, or when you're unable to play?
3. Do you feel the need to play for longer periods of time, play more exciting games, or use more

powerful equipment to get the same amount of excitement you used to get?

4. Have you repeatedly tried to control, cut back, or stop gaming without success?

5. Do you feel less interested in other recreational activities or hobbies because they're not as exciting as gaming?

6. Have you continued gaming even though you knew it was causing problems with your relationships, school or work life, or financial situation?

7. Have you lied to family, friends, or others about how much you game or hid your gaming habits to escape criticism or concern?

8. Do you game to escape from or forget about personal problems, or to relieve uncomfortable feelings such as guilt, anxiety, helplessness or depression?

9. Have you jeopardized or lost significant relationships, a job, or educational or career opportunities because of gaming?

10. Do you feel a sense of relief or comfort when gaming, that you don't feel otherwise?

Add up your score and see where you fall:x

10-20: Gaming seems to be a healthy pastime for you.

21-30: You might have some mild gaming issues, consider keeping an eye on your gaming habits.

31-40: Your gaming habits are edging into the problematic zone. You may want to seek advice or guidance.

41-50: Your responses suggest a likely gaming addiction. It's important to seek help from a mental health professional for further evaluation and possible treatment.

Remember, this self-test is not a replacement for professional diagnosis and treatment. If your gaming is causing problems in your life, seek help regardless of your score.

Violent Games: Understanding and Exploring the Controversy

The digital gaming realm, with its vivid, immersive experiences, can be a double-edged sword, and one area that has received much attention and concern is violent video games and their potential link to aggressive behavior. The debate has been ongoing for years, often rekindled after tragic events, and it is a nuanced and complex issue with differing research perspectives.

The Controversy

The controversy surrounding violent video games and their potential influence on aggression and violence stems from the realistic, interactive nature of many modern games. Unlike passive forms of media, video games often require active engagement, which can include virtual acts of violence in some genres.

The concern is that this virtual violence might desensitize players, especially younger ones, to real-world violence, increase aggressive thoughts and emotions, and decrease pro-social behavior. Moreover, time spent immersed in these games can detract from family time and other vital aspects of social development, potentially increasing feelings of isolation and aggressive behaviors.

The Research Perspectives

Research on this topic has shown mixed results, reflecting the complexity of this issue. Studies have suggested a correlation between playing violent video games and increased aggression in players. They propose that these games can provoke aggressive thoughts, feelings, and physiological responses. They can also decrease prosocial behaviors such as helping and sharing.

Conversely, other studies have found little to no consistent evidence to support these claims. They argue that aggression is influenced by numerous factors, making it challenging to single out video game violence as a primary cause. In fact, some studies have even shown that countries with the highest video game usage often have the lowest societal violence rates.

It's crucial to understand that correlation does not imply causation. While a relationship may exist between violent games and aggression, it does not necessarily mean that one directly causes the other. Factors such as personality traits, family environment, socio-economic status, and others can also play significant roles in the development of aggressive behavior.

Understanding Violence and Aggression

Aggression and violence are not synonymous. Aggression refers to behavior intended to harm another individual, which can be verbal or physical. Violence, on the other hand, refers to extreme forms of aggression, such as physical assault and harm. While some games may increase aggressive thoughts or emotions, this doesn't necessarily translate into violent behavior.

The Role of Parents and Caregivers

Parents and caregivers play a critical role in mitigating potential harmful effects of violent games. They can limit screen time, encourage a balanced mix of activities, monitor the type of games played, and foster open discussions about the difference between gaming realities and real-world consequences.

The Role of Parents in Addressing Gaming and Violence

As a parent, understanding your child's gaming habits and the potential influence of violent content is crucial in the digital age. Your role is more than just a gatekeeper or monitor; it's about being an active participant in their gaming journey.

Why should parents get involved? Because video games are a prominent part of children's culture, and understanding them is an important aspect of connecting with kids and teens. Gaming, like any other hobby, can bring great joy, provide stress relief, and be a legitimate source of skill development. However, just as we protect our children in the real world, we must do so in the digital one.

Research indicates that children and teens, who are in the process of developing their understanding of the world and social norms, are more susceptible to the effects of violent content. Therefore, parental involvement in their gaming experiences is paramount.

Your role can begin with understanding the games your child plays. What is the game's objective? Does it involve violent conflict? If so, how is this violence depicted? Understanding these details can help you have informed conversations with your child about the content they are consuming.

Establishing an open dialogue with your child about their gaming experiences is key. Ask about their games, not with an intention to critique, but to show genuine interest. This can pave the way for discussions about the difference between gaming realities and real-world consequences.

Encourage your child to reflect on their gaming experiences. Ask them how certain games make them feel and what they think about the violence they encounter in their games. By doing this, you are encouraging critical thinking, helping them understand that just because something happens in a game, it doesn't make it acceptable in real life.

Next, set clear expectations and rules about gaming time and the type of games allowed. Explain these rules and the reasoning behind them to your child. Make sure to revisit and adjust these rules as your child grows older and their gaming habits change.

Lastly, educate your child about online safety, especially if they play online games. Explain the risks of sharing personal information and the potential for cyberbullying. Establish guidelines for online interaction and ensure they know what to do if they encounter inappropriate behavior.

Remember, as a parent, your goal isn't to eliminate gaming. Rather, it's to guide your child towards understanding, responsible, and healthy gaming habits. This chapter is not about fearing the digital world, but about understanding its complexities and navigating them wisely. The key is to stay engaged, informed, and maintain open lines of communication with your child. Together, you can turn gaming into a positive and safe digital experience.

Strategies for Preventing and Managing Gaming Addiction

In today's interconnected world, where gaming has become a prevalent form of entertainment, parents and caregivers must grapple with the challenge of managing gaming time and fostering a healthier relationship with digital devices. The potential risk of developing a gaming addiction is real, particularly for the younger generation that has grown up with technology integrated seamlessly into their lives. Understanding this risk and taking proactive steps can help mitigate the adverse effects of excessive gaming.

Set clear boundaries and rules

Start by setting clear boundaries and rules about gaming. This could mean limiting the amount of time your child can play each day or week, setting specific times when gaming is allowed, or designating "gaming-free" zones in your home. It's crucial to establish these rules in collaboration with your child, involving them in the decision-making process to help them feel a sense of ownership and responsibility.

Promote balanced activities

Encourage a range of activities that can balance the sedentary nature of gaming. Physical activity, outdoor play, creative hobbies, reading, and socializing with friends and family in person can provide a healthy counterbalance. A diversified set of activities can also prevent gaming from becoming the primary source of pleasure and entertainment, thereby reducing its addictive potential.

Use parental controls

Most gaming consoles and digital platforms have parental controls that allow you to limit game time, restrict access to certain types of games based on their rating, or even prevent in-game purchases. Utilizing these tools can help ensure your child's gaming experiences are safe and age-appropriate.

Foster open communication

Maintain open lines of communication with your child about their gaming experiences. Ask them about the games they play, who they're playing with, and how they feel during and after gaming. This ongoing dialogue can help you identify any potential issues early on, such as feeling upset when they can't play or if they experience any unpleasant interactions within the game.

Be a role model

Model the balanced digital behavior you want your child to emulate. If they see you using digital devices in a controlled and mindful way, they're likely to follow suit. Remember, your habits—whether it's the amount of time you spend on your phone or how you handle stress—can significantly influence your child's behaviors.

Educate about the risks

Educate your child about the risks of excessive gaming, including its potential impact on their mental and physical health. Explain the concept of gaming addiction and the importance of balance and moderation. The goal is not to instill fear, but to arm them with the knowledge to make informed decisions.

Seek professional help if necessary

If you suspect your child might be developing a gaming addiction—signs could include an obsessive preoccupation with gaming, declining performance in school, withdrawal from other activities, and changes in mood or behavior—don't hesitate to seek professional help. Consult a pediatrician, a child psychologist, or a mental health professional who specializes in digital addiction. Early intervention can make a significant difference in mitigating the impacts of gaming addiction.

Remember, the aim is not to demonize gaming. Video games can offer benefits such as cognitive development, problem-solving skills, and social connection. The key is to promote a balanced, mindful, and healthy approach to gaming. As with many things in life, moderation is crucial. By implementing these strategies, you can help your child navigate the digital landscape responsibly, ensuring that gaming remains a source of enjoyment, not stress or addiction.

Promoting Healthy Gaming Habits

As digital devices become increasingly woven into the fabric of our daily lives, gaming has taken a central role in many young people's leisure time. However, balancing the enjoyment and benefits of gaming with maintaining a healthy lifestyle can be a challenge. This section offers practical suggestions for promoting healthy gaming habits that prioritize balance, physical activity, and time away from screens.

Setting Time Limits

One of the first steps towards promoting healthy gaming habits is setting time limits on gameplay. This helps prevent gaming from taking over too much of your child's day, ensuring that there's enough time left for other activities such as schoolwork, physical exercise, socializing, and downtime. A common approach is to allocate specific 'gaming hours' during the day, perhaps after schoolwork is completed and before bedtime, to avoid sleep disruption.

The key is to involve your child in the decision-making process. Discuss the reason behind setting limits and encourage them to have a say in when their gaming hours should be. This collaborative approach can lead to greater acceptance and adherence to these boundaries.

Encouraging Physical Activity

Regular physical activity is essential for a child's overall health and wellbeing. Encourage your child to engage in a variety of physical activities daily, such as team sports, swimming, biking, or simply playing in the park. It's also worth considering activities that could combine gaming and physical exercise - many consoles offer games designed around physical movement, turning screen time into a fun and engaging workout.

Establishing Gaming-Free Zones and Times

Creating gaming-free zones in your home can help ensure that gaming doesn't encroach on all aspects of family life. This could be as simple as keeping gaming consoles out of bedrooms, ensuring that sleep and relaxation spaces are separate from gaming spaces.

Additionally, designating certain times as 'gaming-free' can be beneficial. This might be during mealtimes, encouraging face-to-face conversation, or in the hour or two before bed, allowing for a 'wind-down' period conducive to good sleep hygiene.

Promoting a Balanced Lifestyle

Help your child maintain a balanced lifestyle, with gaming as just one of many recreational activities. Encourage them to explore other hobbies and interests, spend time outdoors, read books, and engage in creative pursuits. This can help prevent gaming from becoming the sole focus of their free time, reducing the risk of overuse and addiction.

Involvement and Supervision

Take an active interest in the games your child plays. Ask them about their favorite games, who they play with, and what they enjoy about gaming. This can provide valuable insight into their gaming habits and preferences and open up opportunities for discussions around responsible gaming.

Meanwhile, supervision is crucial, particularly for younger children. Make sure you're aware of the games they play and their content. Using parental controls can be an effective way to manage what games they can access and how long they play.

Educating About Safe Online Interactions

Many games today are online, involving interaction with other players worldwide. Teach your child about safe online interactions, emphasizing the importance of not sharing personal information and how to handle inappropriate or uncomfortable situations.

The Value of Offline Relationships

While online friendships formed through gaming can be meaningful, they should not replace offline relationships. Encourage your child to spend time with friends and family offline, promoting face-to-face interactions and real-world experiences.

Promoting healthy gaming habits requires ongoing effort and communication. By setting clear guidelines and promoting a balanced, active lifestyle, you can ensure your child enjoys the benefits of gaming while mitigating potential negative impacts. It's all about balance, supervision, and maintaining open lines of communication.

Strategies: Addressing Cyberbullying in Gaming:

In the vast and dynamic world of online gaming, players connect from all corners of the globe, fostering camaraderie, teamwork, and fun. However, with this connectivity comes an unfortunate dark side—cyberbullying. This section aims to equip you with the knowledge and tools needed to identify and handle cyberbullying within gaming platforms effectively.

Understanding Cyberbullying in Gaming

Cyberbullying in gaming, often termed 'griefing', can range from persistent harassment, spreading rumors, exclusion, to more severe forms like threats and intimidation. It can occur in various ways within a gaming context, such as through in-game chat, personal messages, or even gameplay actions meant to frustrate or humiliate other players. Understanding the different forms cyberbullying can take is the first step towards addressing it.

Prevention Strategies

- Know the Game's Community Standards: Each gaming platform has its own set of community standards or code of conduct that players are expected to adhere to. Familiarize yourself and your child with these standards so that you both understand what behavior is considered acceptable.

- Use Privacy Settings and Controls: Most gaming platforms provide a range of privacy settings and parental controls. Use these tools to manage who can contact your child, who can view their profile, and what kind of content they can access.

- Educate About Online Etiquette and Safety: Teach your child about the importance of treating others with respect online, just as they would in person. Also, stress the significance of not sharing personal information and reporting any inappropriate behavior they encounter.

Recognizing Signs of Cyberbullying

Recognizing the signs of cyberbullying can be challenging as it happens in the digital realm. However, certain behavioral changes may indicate that a child is being cyberbullied. They might become withdrawn, show changes in their gaming habits, appear upset after playing, or start avoiding discussions about their game. They might also exhibit signs of stress or anxiety, have trouble sleeping, or show a decline in academic performance. If you notice such changes, it might be a good time to check in and start a conversation.

Handling Cyberbullying

- Encourage Open Communication: Ensure your child feels comfortable talking about their online experiences, including any instances of cyberbullying. If they've been bullied, remind them it's not their fault and praise their courage for speaking up.

- Document and Report: If your child is being bullied, collect evidence. This could include taking screenshots or noting down details of the incident, like date, time, and the usernames involved. Report the bullying to the game's administrators, who can take appropriate action.

- Block and Report Offenders: Teach your child how to block or mute players who are behaving inappropriately. It's essential they know they have the power to control who they interact with online.

- Seek Support: If your child is affected by cyberbullying, seek help from trusted adults or professional resources. Remember, it's essential to address the emotional impact of cyberbullying alongside tackling the issue itself.

In the end, remember that every gamer has a right to enjoy gaming free from harassment or bullying. As parents, educators, or guardians, it's crucial that we arm our young ones with the knowledge and tools to navigate the gaming world safely and enjoyably.

Research Perspectives: Navigating the Gaming and Violence Discourse

The subject of video games, particularly violent ones, and their impact on players' aggression and behavior has been a topic of passionate debate among researchers, psychologists, and the public alike for decades. This section aims to present an overview of the various viewpoints in this complex discourse, underscoring that the relationship between gaming and violence is nuanced and depends on multiple factors.

The Direct Effects Perspective

One camp in this discussion holds that there is a direct and measurable correlation between exposure to violent video games and increased aggression in players. Several studies seem to support this view. A prominent example is the meta-analysis conducted by Anderson et al., which examined over a hundred studies and concluded that there was indeed a consistent relationship between violent video game exposure and aggressive behavior, angry thoughts, and decreased empathy.

The No Effect Perspective

On the other end of the spectrum, some researchers argue that there's no substantial evidence supporting the idea that violent video games directly contribute to real-world violence or aggression. These researchers point to studies showing that, while there may be a temporary increase in aggression immediately after playing a violent game, there's no evidence that this translates into lasting aggressive behavior in the real world.

The General Aggression Model

The General Aggression Model proposes that violent video games can lead to aggressive behavior, but the impact depends on the individual and the context. For instance, people with a predisposition to aggression or who are in an environment that encourages violence might be more susceptible to the influence of violent games. This approach stresses the importance of individual differences and environmental factors in understanding the impact of violent gaming.

Influence of Game Type and Player Age

The type of game being played and the age of the player also play crucial roles in determining the impact of gaming. Competitive games, even if not violent, may lead to higher levels of aggression due to their competitive nature. On the other hand, cooperative games may reduce aggression and increase pro-social behavior.

The age of the player is another critical factor. Younger children, who are still developing their ability to differentiate between reality and fiction, might be more impressionable to violent content. Conversely, teenagers and adults, who have a better grasp of reality versus fiction, might not be as influenced.

The Moral Panic Argument

Some researchers argue that the controversy surrounding video games and violence is a form of moral panic, similar to the anxieties that arose with the advent of television and rock music. They suggest that the debate might be a social response to the changing media landscape rather than a response to empirical evidence.

The relationship between video games and violent behavior is complex, and the research presents a mixed bag of conclusions. It's essential to consider these varying perspectives and understand that the impact of violent video games is likely to depend on a host of factors, including the individual's personality, their social environment, the nature of the games they play, and how they interact with these games. Rather than seeking a definitive answer to whether games cause violence, perhaps the more practical approach is to guide young gamers towards healthy gaming habits, critical consumption of media, and open conversation about the content they encounter.

Cyberbullying and Online Harassment

Understanding Cyberbullying and Online Harassment

In the digital age, where connectivity is a double-edged sword, cyberbullying and online harassment have become increasingly prominent. To understand this complex issue, it's essential first to define and identify what constitutes these behaviors. Cyberbullying is the use of electronic communication to bully someone, typically by sending messages of an intimidating or threatening nature. Online harassment, a broader term, refers to any unsolicited, often repeated, offensive behavior carried out online. It includes actions like spreading rumors, making threats, or releasing private information about an individual.

The scale and demographics of the problem are alarming. Studies indicate that a significant proportion of internet users, particularly among the younger generation, have experienced some form of online harassment. In the U.S. alone, an estimated 59% of teenagers have experienced cyberbullying, according to a Pew Research Center study. Cyberbullying and online harassment are not confined to any single demographic. They cut across all age groups, genders, races, and socioeconomic statuses. However, teenagers and young adults, given their extensive use of social media platforms, are often more vulnerable.

Different forms of cyberbullying and online harassment exist, each with its distinct characteristics. These include flaming, which involves hostile conversations and name-calling; trolling, which is the act of intentionally provoking or offending others; doxing, the public release of private information; and cyberstalking, the obsessive tracking of a person's online activities. Cyberbullying can also take the form of exclusion or ostracism in online communities, damaging an individual's social connections and sense of belonging.

The prevalence and impact of cyberbullying across age groups and demographics is cause for concern. In children and teenagers, victims of cyberbullying are more likely to experience low self-esteem, poor academic performance, depression, anxiety, and even suicidal thoughts. For adults, the consequences can be equally severe, leading to emotional distress, withdrawal from social connections, and professional repercussions.

In the workplace, online harassment can result in a toxic environment that hampers productivity and job satisfaction. Additionally, cyberbullying and online harassment can exacerbate societal divisions, fueling hate speech, discrimination, and violence. The anonymity offered by the internet often emboldens perpetrators, creating a pervasive sense of insecurity and fear among victims.

The issue of cyberbullying and online harassment is a significant concern in the digital age. It affects a broad spectrum of individuals across various demographics and takes many forms. The impact on victims' mental, emotional, and social well-being is profound. As we move forward in this connected era, it's essential to understand the nature and scale of this problem to develop effective strategies for prevention and intervention. This understanding is the first step towards creating a safer, more respectful online environment for all.

The Psychological Effects of Cyberbullying and Online Harassment

The advent of the internet has revolutionized how we communicate, but it has also opened a new avenue for harm, particularly in the form of cyberbullying and online harassment. This issue is not merely about hurtful comments or messages; it poses severe psychological effects on victims that can have long-term consequences.

One of the immediate impacts of cyberbullying and online harassment is its detrimental effect on mental health and well-being. Victims often experience heightened levels of anxiety and depression. They may also suffer from a significant decrease in self-esteem, leading to feelings of worthlessness and hopelessness. These experiences can be particularly devastating for children and teenagers, whose self-identity and self-worth are still developing.

The anonymity of online platforms can intensify these psychological effects. The victim might feel an overwhelming sense of powerlessness, not knowing who their attacker is or how to protect themselves. The online environment also allows for the constant, inescapable nature of the harassment, creating a chronic state of stress and fear. This persistent anxiety can lead to physical symptoms such as sleep disruption, loss of appetite, and overall declining health.

The long-term consequences of cyberbullying and online harassment are equally concerning. For some victims, the experience can lead to post-traumatic stress disorder (PTSD), a condition usually associated with severe traumatic events. The fear induced by cyberbullying does not necessarily cease when the act stops. Many victims live in ongoing fear of recurrence, causing constant anxiety and vigilance that can hinder their ability to form trusting relationships and engage in social situations.

While it is crucial to understand the psychological effects on victims, it is equally important to acknowledge the role of bystanders and the wider community in addressing cyberbullying. Bystanders who witness cyberbullying incidents are in a unique position to intervene and support the victim. However, they often choose to ignore the incident due to fear of becoming targets themselves or because they believe it's not their business to intervene. This bystander effect can further isolate the victim, adding to their feelings of helplessness and despair.

The wider community also plays a critical role in mitigating the effects of cyberbullying and online harassment. This includes parents, teachers, school administrators, and policymakers. Education about the harmful effects of cyberbullying, coupled with policies and procedures to address it, can create a safer online environment. Providing mental health resources and support for victims is also crucial in helping them cope with the psychological effects.

Cyberbullying and online harassment are not simply problems of the digital age; they are issues of mental health and societal well-being. The psychological impact on victims is profound, with effects ranging from anxiety and depression to post-traumatic stress and ongoing fear. Bystanders and the wider community have a pivotal role to play in combating this issue. Their involvement can make a significant difference, from immediate intervention to long-term prevention strategies. It's a collective responsibility to ensure the internet becomes a safer, more inclusive space for everyone.

Cyberbullying Self-Test

We uncovered the psychological impacts of cyberbullying and online harassment. Such behavior isn't confined merely to playgrounds or workplaces; it can permeate the digital realms we navigate daily. The subtle, often anonymous nature of these interactions can make it challenging to recognize when we've become targets of such behavior.

The following self-test is designed to help us identify possible signs of cyberbullying in our digital interactions. It's important to remember that this test isn't a diagnostic tool, but rather a means to initiate self-awareness and reflection. If any of these questions resonate with your experiences, it may be worth discussing them with a trusted individual or a professional counselor.

For each of the following statements, score yourself as follows:

0 points: I have never experienced this.
1 point: I have rarely experienced this.
2 points: I occasionally experience this.
3 points: I frequently experience this.
Score the following statements from 0-3:

1. I have felt threatened or intimidated by messages I received online.
2. I have been the target of repeated negative comments or ridicule on social media.
3. I have been excluded from an online group or community without reason.
4. Personal, sensitive, or embarrassing information about me has been shared online without my consent.
5. I feel anxiety when receiving notifications or messages from certain individuals or groups.

6. I have been the target of aggressive or harmful behavior online that has persisted despite asking the person to stop.
7. Someone has impersonated me online with the intention of causing harm or embarrassment.
8. I have felt the need to change my online behavior, such as using a different username or deleting my account, because of fear of further harassment.
9. I have felt helpless or hopeless because of something that happened to me online.
10. My offline life (school, work, relationships) has been negatively affected by my online experiences.

Scoring

0-5 points: Low likelihood of being cyberbullied. Your experiences online appear to be generally positive. Remember to maintain healthy online boundaries and stand up for yourself and others when you see or experience negative behavior.

6-15 points: Moderate likelihood of being cyberbullied. Some of your experiences may point to instances of online harassment. It's important to address these issues promptly, by reporting any inappropriate behavior and reaching out to someone you trust for support.

16-30 points: High likelihood of being cyberbullied. Many of your experiences online indicate cyberbullying. It's critical to seek help immediately. Talk to a trusted adult, a counselor, or contact a cyberbullying support service. Remember, you're not alone, and there are many resources available to help you navigate this situation.

The Role of Social Media and Digital Platforms in Cyberbullying

The rise of social media and digital platforms has transformed how we communicate, but it has also led to new avenues for harm. In particular, these platforms have become fertile ground for cyberbullying and online harassment, posing serious concerns for users' safety and well-being.

Social media and other digital platforms have made communication easier and more accessible than ever before. However, these very qualities also make them a breeding ground for cyberbullying. Cyberbullies can hide behind anonymity, making it harder to hold them accountable for their actions. They can target victims around the clock, extending the reach of their harmful actions beyond the physical world into the victim's home and private spaces. Moreover, the permanence of online content means that hurtful posts or messages can continue to cause harm long after they are first published, as they can be viewed and shared repeatedly.

These platforms can also facilitate the rapid spread of harmful content. Cyberbullying incidents can quickly escalate, with rumors, lies, or private information disseminated to a broad audience in mere seconds. The ability to comment, share, or "like" such content can magnify the damage, making the victim feel like they are being attacked by a crowd.

With the power and reach these platforms have, comes a significant level of responsibility. Social media platforms and technology companies play a crucial role in addressing cyberbullying and online harassment. They must establish clear guidelines on acceptable behavior and take swift action against users who violate these rules. They should also provide accessible reporting systems for victims and witnesses of cyberbullying and demonstrate transparency in their handling of such cases. However, there is an ongoing debate over how effectively these platforms are managing this responsibility, with critics arguing they need to do more to protect their users.

While platforms play a crucial role in addressing this issue, it's important not to overlook the role of users and the wider community in preventing cyberbullying. Education about digital literacy and online safety is a crucial part of this. Users, especially young people, need to understand the potential dangers of online interactions and how to protect themselves. They need to know how to recognize cyberbullying, how to report it, and how to support those affected by it.

Digital literacy should also include education about empathy and respectful communication in the digital world. By teaching users to think critically about the potential impact of their online behavior, we can foster a more respectful and inclusive online community.

Social media and digital platforms have a dual nature when it comes to cyberbullying and online harassment. While they can facilitate harmful behavior, they also have the potential to become powerful tools in combating this issue. It requires a combined effort from the platforms themselves, users, and the wider community to create a safer digital environment. Through clear guidelines, effective reporting systems, and digital literacy education, we can reduce the prevalence of cyberbullying and mitigate its harmful effects.

Strategies for Preventing and Addressing Cyberbullying and Online Harassment

The digital era has broadened our horizons, but it has also introduced new forms of harm, such as cyberbullying and online harassment. Dealing with these issues requires a multifaceted approach that combines personal resilience, a supportive network, and promoting a culture of kindness online.

For victims, recognizing and dealing with cyberbullying can be complex. However, some strategies can help. One crucial step is to acknowledge the problem; dismissing or minimizing the issue won't make it go away. If you're a victim, trust your instincts. If someone's words or actions online make you uncomfortable, it's a valid reason to act.

Reporting the issue is the next step. All major social media platforms have mechanisms to report offensive content and abusive behavior. Document everything, taking screenshots or saving communications as evidence. Furthermore, it can be beneficial to confide in someone you trust about what's happening. Emotional support is vital when dealing with such a stressful situation.

Coping strategies can also help mitigate the impact of cyberbullying on mental health. This may include activities that reduce stress and promote well-being, like exercise, meditation, or talking to a mental health professional. It's crucial to remember that you're not alone, and it's not your fault.

Parents, educators, and support networks play a key role in preventing and addressing cyberbullying. They need to foster open communication channels, encouraging children to talk about their online experiences. Parents and educators should be aware of the signs of cyberbullying, which can include changes in mood, behavior, and academic performance. They can also help by promoting responsible internet use and teaching children about the potential risks and consequences of their online behavior.

In schools, anti-cyberbullying programs can help students understand the effects of their actions and equip them with tools to navigate the online world responsibly. Encouraging peer support and bystander intervention can also make a significant impact. Students should be taught to report any incidents of cyberbullying they witness and to support their peers who may be victims.

Promoting empathy, kindness, and positive digital citizenship in the online environment is essential to counter cyberbullying. We need to reinforce the idea that the principles of respect and kindness apply just as much online as they do offline. This includes teaching children from a young age about treating others with respect, not sharing private information without consent, and considering the impact of their words before they post.

In the face of the rising tide of cyberbullying and online harassment, education, access to resources, and the active involvement of bystanders are key to creating safer digital spaces.

Educating users about recognizing and reporting cyberbullying is fundamental. Since digital environments can sometimes blur the lines of acceptable behavior, users must understand what constitutes cyberbullying. This includes recognizing repeated, harmful behaviors such as threats, nasty comments, or spreading rumors online. Users should also know how to use the reporting mechanisms provided by most digital platforms. Encouraging users to report cyberbullying not only helps address the immediate issue but also contributes to the broader effort of creating safe online spaces.

Additionally, users should be aware of the privacy settings available on different platforms. By understanding and applying these settings, we can control who sees our posts and personal information, which can reduce exposure to potential bullies.

Providing tools and resources for victims of cyberbullying is equally crucial. Many organizations offer support services, from counseling to legal advice. Examples include the Cyberbullying Research Center, StopBullying.gov, and the National Suicide Prevention Lifeline, among others. These resources can provide immediate help and long-term strategies for coping with the aftermath of cyberbullying.

There are also numerous apps and tools designed to help combat cyberbullying. These range from apps that detect and filter out offensive content to ones that provide a safe space for victims to share their experiences and receive support. Encouraging victims to utilize these resources can help them regain control of their online experiences.

Empowering bystanders to take an active role in preventing and intervening in instances of cyberbullying can have a profound impact. Bystanders often witness cyberbullying, and their actions can help shape the narrative. When bystanders intervene, they can disrupt the cycle of bullying and provide support to the victim. This can be as simple as sending a private message of support to the victim, reporting the incident, or publicly standing up against the bully.

Educational programs can help empower bystanders by providing them with strategies to intervene effectively without putting themselves at risk. They should also reinforce the importance of not perpetuating bullying, such as by liking, sharing, or commenting on harmful posts.

Strategies for preventing and addressing cyberbullying need to be comprehensive and multifaceted. By educating users, providing tools and resources, and empowering bystanders, we can collectively strive towards making the digital world a safer and more respectful space for everyone. Addressing cyberbullying is a shared responsibility, and each of us has a role to play in this endeavor.

Empowering Parents: Understanding and Addressing Cyberbullying among Children and Teenagers

Throughout the course of this book, we've extensively explored the many facets of our digital lives. Navigating our digital lives can be challenging, especially when it involves protecting our children from potential risks such as cyberbullying.

The digital world, while offering an array of opportunities for learning and connection, is also a platform where bullying can take place in more covert and widespread ways. This phenomenon, known as cyberbullying, can have serious consequences for young minds, potentially impacting their mental health, self-esteem, and academic performance.

One critical aspect is the potential effects of cyberbullying on young minds. These effects can be severe and long-lasting, impacting a child's or teenager's emotional well-being, social interactions, and academic performance. Cyberbullying can lead to feelings of sadness, loneliness, fear, and even depression. In severe cases, it can lead to self-harm or suicidal thoughts. It's crucial to understand these potential effects, as it underlines the importance of timely intervention and support.

Recognizing the signs of cyberbullying is the first step towards intervention. Changes in behavior, mood, or academic performance can signal that something is amiss. For example, a usually outgoing child may become withdrawn, or a high-performing student might start to struggle academically. Similarly, sudden changes in sleep patterns, appetite, or a general lack of interest in activities they once enjoyed can also be red flags.

Another significant sign is an unexplained reluctance to use devices or go online. A child who was once eager to use their digital devices but now avoids them might be experiencing online harassment. We must remember that children and teenagers might not always openly discuss their online experiences due to fear, shame, or a desire to protect their online independence. It's up to us as adults to stay vigilant and approach these situations with understanding and sensitivity.

Understanding the potential effects of cyberbullying and recognizing its signs are crucial steps in protecting our young ones in the digital age. This summary underscores the importance of these insights and encourages us to take a proactive role in safeguarding our children's online experiences. The digital world can be a wonderful place for them to learn, connect, and grow, but only if we ensure it's a safe and respectful environment.

Strategies for Preventing and Addressing Cyberbullying

One of the most effective strategies is promoting open communication about online activities. Regularly talking with our children about their online experiences can help us understand their digital world and the challenges they face. It's essential to foster a safe space where they feel comfortable sharing their online interactions, both positive and negative.

One way to encourage this openness is to take an interest in the digital platforms our children use. This involvement helps us to better understand their online environment and gives us the opportunity to discuss potential risks, including cyberbullying, and ways to handle them.

Another cornerstone of prevention is teaching digital citizenship and empathy. It's crucial for our children to understand that the standards of behavior that apply in the physical world also apply in the digital world. We should instill in them the importance of treating others with respect and kindness online, not sharing private information without consent, and standing up against online harassment when they see it.

Setting clear rules for safe and respectful online behavior is another essential strategy we've highlighted. These rules might include guidelines on sharing personal information, interacting with strangers, and handling negative or abusive online interactions. It's essential that we make these rules together with our children to ensure they understand and agree to them.

Finally, we've discussed using parental controls and monitoring tools responsibly as a part of our strategy. These tools can help us protect our children from inappropriate content and limit their screen time. However, it's important to remember that these tools should complement, not replace, open communication and education about safe online behavior.

Empowering us in understanding and addressing cyberbullying involves a combination of open communication, education, setting clear rules, and the responsible use of parental controls. Each of these strategies plays a vital role in ensuring our children's online experiences are safe and positive. This chapter reiterates the importance of these strategies and encourages us to stay proactive and involved in our children's digital lives. After all, it's not just about protecting them from the risks of the digital world but also about guiding them to use technology in a way that enriches their lives.

Supporting Your Child After a Cyberbullying Incident

Experiencing cyberbullying can be a distressing and traumatic event for our children. It's crucial that we know how to respond effectively to such an incident to reassure and support our child.

The immediate aftermath of a cyberbullying incident is a critical time for providing emotional support and reassurance. We've discussed that it's important to listen to our child's experiences without interruption or judgment, expressing empathy and understanding. It's crucial to validate their feelings and assure them that it's not their fault. We must reinforce the idea that everyone deserves respect, both online and offline.

Moreover, we need to work collaboratively with various entities, such as schools, online platforms, and law enforcement, as necessary. If the bullying involves another student from our child's school, the school administration should be informed and engaged in the process of resolution. Similarly, reporting the abuse to the relevant online platform can lead to the removal of harmful content or even the suspension of the offender's account. In severe cases, when threats or harassment violate the law, we may need to involve law enforcement.

Beyond the immediate response, there's also the long-term support that we can provide to our children. We should monitor for any changes in their behavior or mood that might indicate ongoing distress and consider seeking professional help, such as counseling or therapy, if needed.

Resources for Parents and Families

Finally, as we've explored, there are various resources available for parents and families to support them in dealing with cyberbullying. These resources include websites and hotlines that offer advice, support, and guidance. The Cyberbullying Research Center, StopBullying.gov, and the National Parent Helpline are just a few examples.

Furthermore, a number of books and educational materials can deepen our understanding of cyberbullying and provide strategies for prevention and response. Books like "Bullying Beyond the Schoolyard: Preventing and Responding to Cyberbullying" by Sameer Hinduja and Justin W. Patchin, and "Cyberbullying: What Counselors Need to Know" by Sheri Bauman can be helpful resources.

Supporting our child after a cyberbullying incident requires a combination of emotional support, coordinated response, and long-term vigilance. By utilizing the resources available and maintaining open communication with our child, we can help them recover and build resilience in the face of such adversity.

Legal and Policy Implications of Cyberbullying

The digital landscape has expanded significantly, with cyberbullying and online harassment posing serious challenges. As these issues continue to evolve, so too must our legal frameworks and policies. Understanding the legal consequences, the role of policy and law enforcement, and future directions for legislation and platform policies are key aspects of addressing this growing issue.

The legal consequences of cyberbullying and online harassment vary depending on the jurisdiction. In many countries, such as the United States, the United Kingdom, Canada, and Australia, laws exist that can apply to cases of cyberbullying. These laws often pertain to harassment, stalking, or menacing behavior, and when these actions occur online, we can face serious legal repercussions. It's essential for all of us, especially young internet users, to comprehend that our online actions can have tangible real-world legal consequences.

However, it's worth noting that prosecuting cases of cyberbullying can be challenging due to the often anonymous nature of online interactions and the cross-border nature of the internet. Laws also vary widely by country and even within regions, which can make enforcement difficult.

Policy and law enforcement play a crucial role in addressing cyberbullying and online harassment. Policies set the standards and expectations for behavior in digital spaces, while law enforcement ensures these standards are upheld. Schools, workplaces, and online platforms should have clear policies that define acceptable behavior and outline the consequences for violations. These policies should also detail how incidents should be reported and how they will be handled.

Law enforcement agencies are also evolving to tackle cyberbullying and online harassment more effectively. Many now have dedicated cybercrime units, while others offer training to help officers better understand and address these issues. It's also important that law enforcement agencies work closely with schools, parents, and communities to prevent and respond to cyberbullying incidents.

Looking to the future, legislation and platform policies must continue to adapt to the rapidly changing digital landscape. This may involve updating existing laws to better encompass online behaviors, creating new laws specifically targeting cyberbullying, or increasing the penalties for such actions.

On the platform side, companies must take more responsibility for the content shared on their sites. This could involve stricter enforcement of community guidelines, better reporting mechanisms, and more effective algorithms to detect and remove harmful content. Companies could also collaborate more with external experts, such as mental health professionals and law enforcement agencies, to ensure their policies and procedures are as effective as possible.

Addressing the issue of cyberbullying and online harassment is complex and multifaceted. Legal and policy measures play a vital role, but they must be combined with education, awareness-raising, and support for victims. As our world continues to digitize, it's imperative that we all – policymakers, law enforcement, platform providers, and users alike – work together to make the online world a safer place for everyone.

The Effects of Technology On Sleep And Physical Health

The Science of Sleep and Technology's Impact

Sleep, an integral part of human life, is a fascinating subject that's been extensively researched by scientists across the globe. It's not simply a period of rest, but a dynamic process that involves numerous biological and physiological functions, vital for overall health and well-being. We will delve into the science of sleep, focusing particularly on the implications of technology use on our sleep patterns and quality.

To start with, it's crucial to understand the sleep cycle, a repeated pattern of sleep stages occurring throughout the night. Sleep is primarily composed of two distinct types: Rapid Eye Movement (REM) sleep, where most dreaming occurs, and Non-Rapid Eye Movement (NREM) sleep, further divided into three stages — N1, N2, and N3. Stage N3 is what we commonly refer to as 'deep sleep.' These stages cycle approximately every 90 minutes, with periods of REM sleep becoming longer as the night progresses. A good night's sleep ideally consists of multiple cycles of these stages, allowing us to wake up feeling refreshed and rejuvenated.

However, our digital habits can disrupt this natural rhythm. One of the primary culprits is blue light, a type of light emitted by the screens of our digital devices such as smartphones, tablets, computers, and TVs. While our exposure to blue light during daylight hours can be beneficial, helping us stay alert and improving our mood and cognitive performance, exposure during the evening can have a detrimental effect on our sleep.

Blue light interferes with the production of melatonin, a hormone secreted by the pineal gland in the brain, which signals to our bodies that it's time to sleep. As darkness falls, our melatonin levels naturally rise, reaching a peak in the late evening and remaining high throughout the night. However, exposure to blue light from screens can trick our brains into thinking it's still daylight, suppressing the production of melatonin, delaying sleep onset, and disrupting our sleep-wake cycle.

The impact of digital devices on sleep extends beyond blue light exposure. The constant connectivity that our devices offer can lead to increased stress and anxiety, further affecting sleep quality and quantity. Receiving work emails late into the night, engaging in emotionally-charged conversations on social media, or even just the anticipation of these notifications can trigger a stress response, making it difficult to unwind and fall asleep.

Moreover, the stimulating content available online can cause cognitive arousal, making our minds too active for sleep. Whether it's an intense episode of a TV series, an engaging video game, or a deep dive into a rabbit hole of online information, these activities can cause us to delay our bedtime, reducing the total hours of sleep we get.

Understanding the implications of technology use on our sleep is the first step towards making positive changes. By being mindful of our screen habits, particularly in the hours leading up to bedtime, we can reduce the impact of technology on our sleep and improve our overall health and well-being.

We'll also discuss various strategies to manage our digital habits and promote better sleep, such as establishing a digital curfew, using night mode features on our devices, and creating a sleep-friendly environment. By implementing these strategies, we can harness the benefits of technology while minimizing its potential negative impacts on our sleep and overall health.

Physical Health Consequences of Excessive Screen Time

The proliferation of digital technology in our daily lives, while undoubtedly beneficial, has also led to an increase in sedentary behavior and its associated health risks. Long hours in front of screens, whether for work or leisure, can have far-reaching implications for our physical health, impacting everything from our posture to our eyes. We will delve into some of these consequences, examining the physical toll of excessive screen time.

Sedentary behavior, characterized by activities that require minimal physical effort and involve sitting or reclining, is a growing concern in our technology-driven society. The time we spend seated in front of screens is time we are not spending on physical activity, contributing to an overall sedentary lifestyle. Sedentary behavior has been linked with numerous health concerns, including obesity, cardiovascular disease, and type 2 diabetes. Research also suggests that high levels of sedentary time could be associated with an increased risk of certain cancers. Moreover, a sedentary lifestyle can lead to muscle atrophy and weakening, particularly in the lower body, resulting in reduced functional fitness and mobility.

Beyond its contribution to a sedentary lifestyle, excessive screen time can also directly impact our musculoskeletal health, particularly our posture. Prolonged sitting, often in ergonomically poor positions, coupled with the tendency to lean forward towards our screens, can lead to postural imbalances and musculoskeletal discomfort. This 'tech neck' or 'forward head posture' can lead to chronic neck and shoulder pain, tension headaches, and even long-term damage to the cervical spine. Additionally, the repetitive use of handheld devices can contribute to conditions such as carpal tunnel syndrome and tendonitis in the hands and wrists.

Another major health concern associated with extensive screen time is eye strain, technically referred to as asthenopia. Symptoms of eye strain include dry or watery eyes, blurred vision, sensitivity to light, and headaches. Extended periods of screen use can exacerbate these symptoms, leading to a condition known as digital eye strain or computer vision syndrome. The blue light emitted from screens can also contribute to digital eye strain and potentially harm the light-sensitive cells in the retina.

But the aim here isn't to stoke fear or advocate for the complete abandonment of technology. Rather, the goal is to promote awareness and encourage mindful tech use. There are practical measures we can take to mitigate these risks, such as using ergonomically designed workstations, taking frequent screen breaks, practicing regular physical activity, and following the 20-20-20 rule for our eyes (every 20 minutes, look at something 20 feet away for at least 20 seconds).

We'll dive deeper into strategies for managing screen time and promoting physical health, such as incorporating movement into our day, practicing good posture, and taking steps to prevent digital eye strain. By making these small but significant changes, we can enjoy the conveniences of technology without compromising our physical health.

Navigating the digital world with intention and balance involves a holistic approach, considering not just the psychological implications of our digital habits, but also their physical health consequences. As we move forward in this digital age, let's remember to prioritize our health and well-being, taking the necessary steps to foster a healthier relationship with technology.

The Intersection of Mental Health and Physical Well-being

The interplay between mental health and physical well-being is a fundamental aspect of human health, a relationship that becomes even more pronounced in the context of our digital lives. With the pervasiveness of technology and the consequent physical and mental health implications, a comprehensive understanding of this intersection is crucial.

Poor sleep and physical health issues, common consequences of excessive screen time, can further aggravate mental health concerns. Sleep is a restorative process, playing a vital role in cognitive functioning, emotional regulation, and overall health. A disruption in sleep patterns, often induced by the blue light emitted from screens, can lead to daytime fatigue, reduced cognitive performance, and mood disturbances, escalating existing mental health conditions such as anxiety and depression. Chronic sleep deprivation can even increase the risk of developing these conditions.

Physical health issues stemming from a sedentary lifestyle, such as obesity and cardiovascular disease, can also contribute to poor mental health. The interplay of chronic physical conditions and mental health is complex and bidirectional, with each having the potential to adversely affect the other. For instance, chronic pain or discomfort resulting from poor posture can lead to increased stress, anxiety, or feelings of depression, which in turn can further worsen the physical condition.

In the digital age, a holistic approach to well-being becomes increasingly critical. This approach acknowledges the intricate connection between the mind and the body, emphasizing the importance of addressing both physical and mental health to achieve overall well-being. It's not just about managing screen time or promoting physical activity; it's also about fostering mental resilience, managing stress, and maintaining a positive attitude towards personal growth and self-improvement.

Implementing strategies that address both mental and physical health simultaneously is an integral part of this holistic approach. Regular physical activity is one such strategy. It promotes better sleep, helps maintain a healthy weight, and also acts as a natural mood booster, reducing symptoms of depression and anxiety.

Mindfulness practices can also have dual benefits. By focusing on the present moment, we can reduce stress and anxiety while also becoming more aware of our physical state, allowing us to identify and address any physical discomfort or tension early on.

Creating a balanced and healthy relationship with technology is another key strategy. This involves setting boundaries around tech use, taking regular breaks, and practicing digital detox. Not only can these measures reduce the risk of physical health issues such as eye strain and postural problems, but they can also help to mitigate the risk of technology-induced stress, anxiety, and depression.

We'll also look into these strategies, providing practical tips and techniques to maintain both your mental and physical health in the face of increasing digital demands. We'll explore how to cultivate a growth mindset, set healthy boundaries with technology, and develop a routine that promotes both physical and mental well-being. By combining these strategies, we can navigate the digital world in a way that prioritizes and protects our overall health.

The intersection of mental health and physical well-being is an area that requires our attention and care. As we continue to embrace digital technology, let's ensure we do so in a way that honors both our minds and bodies, promoting a holistic sense of well-being.

Strategies for Healthy Sleep and Physical Health in the Digital Age

As the digital era evolves, so must our strategies for maintaining our health. Healthy sleep and physical well-being are integral to our overall health, and yet, they can be negatively impacted by excessive screen time and a sedentary lifestyle. Here are some practical tips for promoting healthy sleep and physical health in the digital age.

Starting with sleep, establishing a consistent sleep schedule and bedtime routine is key. Our bodies thrive on consistency, and setting a fixed time for sleeping and waking up can help regulate our internal body clock, also known as the circadian rhythm. This routine signals to our body when it's time to sleep and wake up, leading to better sleep quality and daytime alertness. A calming bedtime routine can further enhance this. This routine might include reading a physical book, practicing light stretching, or other relaxing activities that don't involve screens.

Creating a sleep-friendly environment free from digital distractions is also important. The blue light emitted from screens can interfere with the production of melatonin, the hormone that regulates sleep. To mitigate this, consider removing electronic devices from your bedroom or using apps that filter out blue light. Make your sleeping space quiet, dark, and cool, and invest in a comfortable mattress and pillows. These changes can make a significant difference to the quality of your sleep.

Physical activity is another pillar of good health that can be easily overlooked in our increasingly digital lives. Incorporating physical activity and exercise into daily routines is essential. This doesn't necessarily mean hitting the gym every day; it could involve taking short breaks to stretch or walk around during the workday, taking the stairs instead of the elevator, or participating in a sport or activity you enjoy. Regular exercise has numerous benefits, from promoting better sleep and reducing the risk of chronic diseases to enhancing mood and cognitive function.

Finally, promoting a more balanced relationship with technology can significantly contribute to better sleep and physical health. Here are a few tips for reducing screen time:

1. Set boundaries: Establish set times during the day when you are free from digital devices. This could be during meals, the hour before bed, or during family time.

2. Use technology to your advantage: Utilize apps and settings that track and limit your screen time or remind you to take breaks.

3. Be selective: Not all screen time is created equal. Be selective about the digital content you consume. Aim for quality over quantity.

4. Engage in offline activities: Allocate time for offline activities that you enjoy. This could be anything from reading, painting, cooking, or spending time in nature.

While the digital age brings with it many conveniences, it also presents challenges to our sleep and physical health. By implementing these practical tips, you can foster healthy sleep habits, enhance your physical well-being, and cultivate a more balanced relationship with technology. As we navigate through the digital age, let's do so with a commitment to our overall health and well-being.

Building Digital Resilience

Understanding Digital Resilience

In an era where technology is interwoven into every aspect of life, the ability to navigate the digital world while maintaining mental health and well-being has become critical. This ability, known as digital resilience, is not just about avoiding online dangers, but also about knowing how to handle them when they arise, and using technology in a positive and productive way.

Digital resilience is a multifaceted concept that includes emotional, cognitive, and behavioral components. It involves having the emotional strength to withstand and bounce back from the challenges of the online world, such as cyberbullying, online harassment, or digital addiction. It also includes the cognitive skills to understand the nature of these challenges, discern the real from the fake, and make informed decisions about online behavior. Lastly, it involves the behavioral ability to implement protective strategies, such as setting boundaries around technology use, practicing digital detox, and using online resources for support and help when needed.

Digital resilience is of paramount importance in the digital age. As technology continues to evolve, the challenges and risks associated with it also grow. Cyberbullying, online harassment, digital addiction, and the spread of misinformation are just a few of the issues that can affect our mental health and well-being.By collectively fostering digital resilience, we can navigate these challenges more effectively, minimizing negative impacts and fostering healthier online experiences.

Moreover, digital resilience can help us to harness the positive potential of technology. With resilience, we are better equipped to leverage technology for learning, creativity, connection, and support. They can take advantage of the wealth of resources available online while minimizing the potential drawbacks.

There are several benefits of digital resilience for mental health and well-being. Firstly, it can help to prevent or reduce the impact of online-related stress and anxiety. By knowing how to handle online challenges, we can feel more confident and less anxious about their online interactions. Secondly, digital resilience can foster a healthier relationship with technology, reducing the risk of digital addiction and its associated negative effects on mental health.

Thirdly, digital resilience can empower us to use technology as a tool for support and self-improvement. Many resources, from mental health apps to online support groups, can be leveraged to enhance mental health and well-being. Lastly, digital resilience can promote overall personal growth and development. By facing and overcoming online challenges, we can develop important life skills, such as problem-solving, critical thinking, and emotional intelligence.

Building digital resilience is a vital task in the digital age. It's a protective shield that allows us to navigate the complexities of the online world, mitigating risks and maximizing benefits. By understanding and fostering digital resilience, we can equip ourselves and others to thrive in an increasingly digital world.

Developing Emotional Resilience in the Digital World

In an era where technology is interwoven into every aspect of life, the ability to navigate the digital world while maintaining mental health and well-being has become critical. This ability, known as digital resilience, is not just about avoiding online dangers, but also about knowing how to handle them when they arise, and using technology in a positive and productive way.

Digital resilience is a multifaceted concept that includes emotional, cognitive, and behavioral components. It involves having the emotional strength to withstand and bounce back from the challenges of the online world, such as cyberbullying, online harassment, or digital addiction. It also includes the cognitive skills to understand the nature of these challenges, discern the real from the fake, and make informed decisions about online behavior. Lastly, it involves the behavioral ability to implement protective strategies, such as setting boundaries around technology use, practicing digital detox, and using online resources for support and help when needed.

Digital resilience is of paramount importance in the digital age. As technology continues to evolve, the challenges and risks associated with it also grow. Cyberbullying, online harassment, digital addiction, and the spread of misinformation are just a few of the issues that can affect our mental health and well-being. By developing digital resilience, we can better navigate these challenges, reducing their negative impact and promoting healthier online experiences.

Moreover, digital resilience can help us to harness the positive potential of technology. With resilience, we are better equipped to leverage technology for learning, creativity, connection, and support. They can take advantage of the wealth of resources available online while minimizing the potential drawbacks.

There are several benefits of digital resilience for mental health and well-being. Firstly, it can help to prevent or reduce the impact of online-related stress and anxiety. By knowing how to handle online challenges, we can feel more confident and less anxious about our online interactions. Secondly, digital resilience can foster a healthier relationship with technology, reducing the risk of digital addiction and its associated negative effects on mental health.

Thirdly, digital resilience can empower us to use technology as a tool for support and self-improvement. Many resources, from mental health apps to online support groups, can be leveraged to enhance mental health and well-being. Lastly, digital resilience can promote overall personal growth and development. By facing and overcoming online challenges, we can develop important life skills, such as problem-solving, critical thinking, and emotional intelligence.

Building digital resilience is a vital task in the digital age. It's a protective shield that allows us to navigate the complexities of the online world, mitigating risks and maximizing benefits. By understanding and fostering digital resilience, we can equip ourselves and others to thrive in an increasingly digital world.

Enhancing Cognitive Resilience in the Digital Age

In the digital age, cognitive resilience is vital for managing and adapting to the constant flux of information, platforms, and technologies. We will dive into strategies for enhancing cognitive resilience by fostering critical thinking, adaptability, and balancing online and offline experiences.

Critical thinking and discernment are essential tools in online information consumption. The digital landscape is brimming with data - not all of it accurate or beneficial. Our ability to assess, analyze, and make informed decisions about this information is vital. This requires questioning sources, comparing perspectives, recognizing biases, and discerning fact from fiction. It's about developing a keen digital discernment, allowing us to navigate online spaces with a critical eye and an informed mind. This helps us protect ourselves from misinformation, digital scams, or content that may be harmful to our well-being.

A growth mindset, first proposed by psychologist Carol Dweck, refers to the belief that our abilities, intelligence, and skills can be developed over time through effort and practice. This mindset is a key component of cognitive resilience in the digital age. With technology continually evolving, we face a constant stream of new platforms, tools, and digital challenges. Viewing these challenges as opportunities for learning and growth, rather than threats or obstacles, can help us adapt more effectively. This mindset encourages us to embrace the digital landscape as a dynamic learning environment, boosting our confidence and resilience in the face of digital change.

Balancing online and offline experiences is another important aspect of cognitive resilience. While the digital world offers numerous opportunities for learning, entertainment, and connection, it's also essential to engage in offline activities that stimulate our cognitive abilities in different ways. This might include reading a physical book, solving a puzzle, engaging in meaningful face-to-face conversations, or immersing ourselves in nature. These activities can provide a restorative break from screen time, support diverse cognitive functions, and enhance our overall cognitive resilience.

Moreover, offline experiences can provide opportunities for reflection and consolidation of online learning. They can offer fresh perspectives and inspire new ideas, contributing to a more holistic and balanced cognitive experience. It's about recognizing that while the digital world is a powerful cognitive tool, it's not the only one at our disposal.

Enhancing cognitive resilience in the digital age involves developing critical thinking skills, cultivating a growth mindset, and balancing online and offline experiences. These strategies can equip us to navigate the digital world with an open, adaptive mind, turning digital disruptions into opportunities for cognitive growth and development. As digital citizens, it's about not just surviving in the digital age, but thriving, and cognitive resilience is a key part of that journey.

Strengthening Behavioral Resilience in the Digital Environment

As our reliance on digital technologies continues to grow, developing behavioral resilience in the digital environment becomes increasingly crucial. We will discuss strategies for establishing healthy digital habits, incorporating digital detoxes, mindful technology use, and leveraging support networks and professional help when needed.

Establishing healthy digital habits and boundaries is the first step toward building behavioral resilience in the digital environment. This involves being intentional about our technology use, setting clear boundaries around screen time, and prioritizing activities that contribute to our overall well-being. For instance, we can create a designated 'tech-free' time during the day, refrain from using devices during meals or before bedtime, and use technology in a way that aligns with our personal values and goals. It's about making conscious choices that support our mental and physical health, relationships, productivity, and leisure.

Digital detox, or consciously reducing or eliminating screen time for a specific period, is an effective strategy for fostering behavioral resilience. A digital detox can help us reset our digital habits, reduce dependency on devices, and create space for engaging in other enriching activities. This could be as simple as a one-hour break from screens each day, a tech-free weekend, or a more extended period of digital disconnection. The key is to find a balance that works for you and aligns with your lifestyle and needs.

Mindful technology use, a concept we touched on earlier, is another essential aspect of behavioral resilience. This means being fully present and intentional in our digital interactions, using technology as a tool rather than letting it dictate our behavior. It involves noticing how we're engaging with technology, how it makes us feel, and making adjustments as necessary. Mindfulness can help us break free from autopilot scrolling, reduce digital distractions, and foster a more balanced and fulfilling digital experience.

Finally, building support networks and seeking professional help when needed are vital components of behavioral resilience in the digital environment. Friends, family, and communities can provide emotional support, share strategies for managing digital challenges, and offer a sense of belonging and connection. If we're struggling with issues such as digital addiction or cyberbullying, professional help, such as counseling or therapy, can provide specialized support and interventions. There are also numerous online resources and platforms that offer support and guidance for managing digital challenges.

Strengthening behavioral resilience in the digital environment involves a combination of healthy digital habits, digital detoxes, mindful technology use, and leveraging support networks and professional resources. By adopting these strategies, we can navigate the digital world with resilience, maintaining our well-being in the face of digital challenges and making the most of the opportunities that technology has to offer.

Strategies & Tips for Building Digital Resilience

As we continue to immerse ourselves in the digital world, building digital resilience becomes imperative to maintain our mental and physical well-being. It is a multidimensional approach that involves mindful self-reflection, setting realistic digital engagement goals, and fostering open communication about our digital experiences.

Incorporating self-reflection and mindfulness practices into our daily routines is a powerful strategy for building digital resilience. Self-reflection allows us to pause and assess our digital habits: What apps or websites do we spend the most time on? How do we feel during and after using these platforms? Do these activities align with our values and goals? By asking these questions, we can gain a clearer understanding of our digital behaviors and make necessary adjustments to support our well-being.

Mindfulness, the practice of paying deliberate attention to the present moment without judgment, can also enhance our digital resilience. For example, we can incorporate mindfulness into our technology use by noticing the sensations, thoughts, and emotions that arise during our digital interactions. We can take a few moments to focus on our breath before responding to an email or a comment online, bringing a sense of calm and clarity to our digital communications.

Setting realistic goals and expectations for digital engagement is another important aspect of building digital resilience. This involves being clear about why we're using digital technologies and what we hope to achieve through our digital interactions. It's about recognizing that while technology can offer many benefits, it's not a panacea for all our needs and challenges. For example, social media can help us stay connected with friends and family, but it's not a substitute for face-to-face interactions and meaningful offline experiences. By setting realistic expectations, we can use technology in a way that enhances our lives while mitigating potential drawbacks.

Encouraging open communication and discussion around digital experiences and challenges is crucial for fostering digital resilience. This can involve sharing our own experiences, listening to others' perspectives, and offering mutual support. For parents and educators, it's about creating a safe and supportive environment where children and young people can express their thoughts and feelings about their online experiences, ask questions, and learn from each other. For adults, it could involve participating in online forums or support groups focused on digital well-being, or discussing digital habits and challenges with friends, family, or a mental health professional.

As we delve deeper into the realm of digital resilience, the importance of enhancing digital literacy and fostering critical thinking becomes increasingly clear. These abilities are critical in the current digital landscape, where misinformation abounds and online interactions can have real-world implications.

Digital literacy is no longer a luxury but a necessity in today's interconnected world. It encompasses a broad set of skills including, but not limited to, understanding how digital technologies work, using them effectively, and being aware of the ethical and societal issues related to their use. Here are some practical ways to improve your digital literacy:

1. Engage in Continuous Learning: The digital landscape is continuously evolving, and staying updated requires constant learning. Participate in online courses, webinars, or workshops focused on enhancing digital skills. Resources like MOOCs (Massive Open Online Courses) offer free courses on a wide array of digital literacy topics.

2. Practice Safe Online Behavior: Protecting yourself and others online is a crucial aspect of digital literacy. This involves understanding the importance of online privacy and security, using strong, unique passwords for different accounts, and being cautious when sharing personal information online.

3. Understand Digital Etiquette: Digital literacy also includes understanding and adhering to digital etiquette or 'netiquette'. This involves respecting others' opinions online, avoiding cyberbullying, and understanding the impact of your digital footprint.

Critical thinking is another vital component of digital resilience. It empowers us to evaluate the credibility of online information, discern fact from fiction, and make informed decisions about our online interactions. Here are some tips to foster critical thinking in the digital age:

1. Check the Source: Before sharing or acting upon online information, always consider the source. Is it a reputable news outlet, an expert in the field, or a trusted organization? If not, the information may be unreliable or misleading.

2. Look for Evidence: Don't accept information at face value. Look for evidence that supports the claims being made. This could involve checking multiple sources or conducting your own research.

3. Think Before You Click: Before clicking on links or downloading files, think about the potential consequences. Could the link lead to a malicious website? Could the file contain a virus? If in doubt, don't click.

4. Reflect on Your Biases: We all have biases that can influence how we interpret and respond to information. By acknowledging these biases, we can strive to view online content more objectively and make more balanced decisions.

By enhancing our digital literacy skills and fostering critical thinking, we can better navigate online spaces, protect ourselves from digital threats, and contribute to a healthier and more respectful digital environment. This, in turn, strengthens our overall digital resilience, enabling us to thrive in the digital age.

Building digital resilience is a proactive and ongoing process that involves self-reflection, setting realistic digital engagement goals, and fostering open communication about our digital experiences. These strategies can empower us to navigate the digital world with confidence and resilience, supporting our overall well-being in the digital age.

Empowering Digital Resilience in Self and Others

Empowering Digital Resilience in Self and Others

Digital resilience is not only a personal journey but a collective one. As we learn to navigate the digital world with increased consciousness and adaptability, it becomes equally important to empower others to do the same.

Role Modeling Digital Resilience in Personal and Professional Networks

The first step towards empowering others is to model the behavior we want to see. As we become more digitally resilient, we can set an example for our family members, friends, colleagues, and others in our network. Here are some ways we can do this:

1. Maintain Healthy Digital Habits: Be conscious of your screen time and make sure to balance it with offline activities. Make it a point to detach from your digital devices during meals, before bedtime, and when spending time with loved ones. Others may follow suit when they see the benefits of these habits.

2. Promote Mindful Tech Use: Talk about your experiences with mindful technology use. Share the strategies that have worked for you in dealing with digital distractions, online negativity, or information overload.

3. Encourage Open Communication: Be open about the challenges you face in the digital world. This can help others feel more comfortable discussing their own experiences and concerns, fostering a more supportive and understanding environment.

4. Set Boundaries: Demonstrate how you set boundaries with technology, such as designated tech-free times or spaces in your home, or turning off non-essential notifications. This can inspire others to consider their own digital boundaries.

Collaborating to Create a More Resilient Digital Society

We can make a difference, but collectively, we can transform the digital landscape. Here are some ways we can collaborate to create a more resilient digital society:

1. Promote Digital Literacy: Whether you're a parent, educator, or a community leader, you can help others understand the importance of digital literacy. Encourage schools and community centers to incorporate digital literacy in their curriculum and programs.

2. Support Policies that Promote Digital Wellness: Advocate for policies that protect digital rights and promote digital wellness, such as laws against cyberbullying, or company policies that respect digital boundaries and prevent digital overload.

3. Support Initiatives that Foster Digital Resilience: Participate in and support initiatives that aim to build digital resilience, such as workshops, campaigns, or online communities focused on digital well-being.

4. Foster a Positive Digital Culture: Encourage empathy, respect, and positivity in online interactions. Stand against online harassment and misinformation, and support victims of cyberbullying.

Empowering digital resilience in ourselves and others is a powerful step towards creating a healthier, more balanced digital world. By role modeling resilient behaviors and collaborating for a more resilient society, we can ensure that the digital age is an age of opportunity, connection, and well-being for all.

Digital Minimalism And Detoxification

Understanding Digital Minimalism and Detoxification

In a world where digital connectivity is constant, the concept of digital minimalism and detoxification emerges as a refreshing antidote. We will delve into the principles and benefits of digital minimalism and detoxification, their positive impacts on mental health and well-being, and the philosophy behind choosing this lifestyle.

Defining Digital Minimalism and Detoxification, Principles and Benefits

Digital Minimalism is a philosophy that encourages a more mindful and intentional use of technology. It is not about completely eliminating digital devices from our lives, but rather about optimizing their usage to add value and reduce distractions. The basic principle is to use technology as a tool to support our goals and values, rather than letting it dictate our time and attention.

Digital detoxification, on the other hand, is a temporary break or retreat from digital devices. The duration can vary from a few hours in a day to a few days or weeks. The goal of a digital detox is to provide an opportunity to disconnect, recharge, and evaluate our relationship with technology.

The benefits of digital minimalism and detoxification are manifold. They can help:

1. Reduce Anxiety and Stress: Constant connectivity can lead to increased anxiety and stress. Digital minimalism and detoxification can help us disconnect, relax, and reduce stress levels.

2. Improve Focus and Productivity: By reducing digital distractions, we can improve our focus and productivity in both our professional and personal lives.

3. Enhance Relationships: By being more present and less distracted, we can improve our relationships with others.

4. Promote Better Sleep: Reducing screen time, especially before bed, can improve sleep quality.

The Philosophy Behind Digital Minimalism as a Lifestyle Choice

At its core, digital minimalism is a conscious and deliberate approach to our digital lives. It is a lifestyle choice that emphasizes quality over quantity, where we choose to engage with technology in a way that supports our personal and professional goals, rather than detracting from them.

The philosophy behind digital minimalism is centered around three key principles:

1. Clarity of Purpose: Digital minimalists are clear about why they are using technology. They use it as a tool to support their values and what they care about most, rather than using it in a mindless or habitual way.

2. Intentionality: Digital minimalists are intentional about their technology use. They make deliberate decisions about what technologies to use, how to use them, and when to use them. They don't simply accept every digital tool that comes their way; they assess each one for its real value and potential drawbacks.

3. Mindfulness: Digital minimalists use technology mindfully. They are present in their digital interactions and use technology in a way that aligns with their mental and emotional well-being.

Adopting a digital minimalist lifestyle doesn't mean renouncing all digital technologies. On the contrary, it's about making more mindful, intentional choices about how we use these tools. It's about finding the right balance between connectivity and disconnection, so that we can reap the benefits of digital technology without letting it overtake our lives.

Implementing Digital Minimalism Principles

Recognizing Signs of Digital Overload and Its Impact on Well-being

In our increasingly connected world, it's easy to find ourselves overwhelmed by the constant barrage of information, notifications, and digital demands. This digital overload can lead to various negative impacts on our mental and physical well-being. It can disrupt our sleep, increase stress, decrease productivity, impair our social relationships, and generally reduce our quality of life.

Recognizing the signs of digital overload is the first step towards implementing digital minimalism principles. These signs can vary from person to person, but common symptoms include feeling anxious or stressed when separated from your devices, compulsive checking of social media or emails, spending more time online than intended, and neglecting other important aspects of life, such as physical health, relationships, or work responsibilities.

Another sign is a general sense of dissatisfaction or frustration with your digital habits, or feeling that your digital life is out of control. You may also find that your digital activities are not adding value to your life, but are instead distracting you from your real-life goals and values.

Evaluating Personal Technology Use and Identifying Areas for Change

Once you have recognized the signs of digital overload, the next step is to evaluate your personal technology use. This involves taking an honest look at your digital habits and asking yourself some hard questions. Which digital activities are truly beneficial to you, and which ones are merely wasting your time or causing stress? Are there any specific apps or websites that are particularly problematic for you?

One useful approach is to keep a digital diary for a week or two, noting down how much time you spend on different digital activities and how these activities make you feel. This can give you a clearer picture of your digital habits and help you identify areas for change.

Decluttering Digital Devices and Applications

Decluttering your digital devices and applications is a key part of digital minimalism. This means deleting unnecessary apps, turning off non-essential notifications, and organizing your digital files and documents.

Start by going through all your digital devices - smartphone, tablet, laptop - and remove any apps or files that you don't use or need. This can free up mental space and reduce distractions, making it easier to focus on the digital activities that truly matter to you.

Next, consider which notifications you really need. Many of us allow apps to send us notifications without considering whether they are truly necessary. Turn off any notifications that aren't essential or beneficial to your life.

Decluttering your digital environment can be a liberating experience. It can help you regain control over your digital life, reduce feelings of overwhelm, and make your digital experiences more enjoyable and productive. Remember, the goal of digital minimalism is not to eliminate all digital activities, but to ensure that the ones you engage in are truly beneficial and align with your personal goals and values.

Intentional Technology Use and Mindful Engagement with Digital Content

As we become more aware of our digital habits, it's crucial to shift from mindless to mindful engagement with technology. Intentional technology use means consciously deciding what role digital devices and online platforms will play in our lives. It's about using technology as a tool to serve our needs and values, rather than letting it control us.

Mindful engagement with digital content involves being present and focused when using technology. Instead of passively scrolling through social media feeds or multitasking across multiple tabs, we give our full attention to one task or piece of content at a time. This can increase our enjoyment and understanding of the content, reduce feelings of overwhelm, and help us make more deliberate choices about our digital activities.

Reducing Digital Distractions and Prioritizing High-Value Online Activities

To implement digital minimalism principles, it's important to reduce digital distractions and prioritize high-value online activities. Digital distractions can come in many forms, from incessant notifications and emails to the endless scroll of social media feeds. These distractions can fragment our attention, impair our productivity, and increase our stress levels.

To reduce digital distractions, we can set boundaries for our technology use. This might involve designated tech-free times or zones, using website or app blockers, or disabling notifications during focused work periods. It's also helpful to prioritize high-value online activities - those that genuinely enrich our lives, align with our goals, or provide essential services.

Strategies for Adopting a Minimalist Approach to Technology Use

Adopting a minimalist approach to technology use can be a gradual process. Here are some strategies to guide you:

- Start Small: Begin with one aspect of your digital life that you'd like to change, such as reducing your social media use or decluttering your email inbox. Once you've made progress in this area, you can tackle other aspects.

- Establish Clear Goals: Having clear, concrete goals can help motivate you and keep you on track. For instance, you might aim to spend no more than an hour a day on social media, or to check your emails only at specific times.

- Create Tech-Free Spaces and Times: Designate certain spaces in your home (such as the bedroom or dining room) as tech-free zones, and certain times of the day (such as the first hour after waking or the hour before bed) as tech-free times.

- Use Tools to Help: There are various tools and apps available to help you reduce digital distractions and manage your technology use, such as website or app blockers, time tracking apps, and digital wellbeing features on your devices.

- Seek Support: Let your friends and family know about your digital minimalism journey, and consider seeking their support. You might even inspire them to join you!

Remember, the goal of digital minimalism isn't to eliminate technology from our lives, but to use it in a way that supports our well-being and aligns with our values. It's about making conscious, intentional choices, and reclaiming our time and attention from the digital distractions that so often consume them.

Strategies for Digital Detoxification

A digital detox is a period of time during which we voluntarily refrain from using digital devices like smartphones, computers, and social media platforms. Planning a successful digital detox requires some thought and preparation. Here are some steps you can follow:

1. Define your objectives: What do you hope to achieve through your digital detox? Whether it's to reduce stress, improve concentration, spend more time on offline activities, or improve sleep, having clear objectives can help keep you motivated.

2. Decide on the duration and scope of your detox: Will it be a complete break from all digital devices for a day or a week, or a partial detox restricting only certain platforms or activities?

3. Prepare in advance: Notify friends, family, and colleagues about your planned digital detox. If you're planning a longer detox, you might need to set up auto-responses on your email or other communication platforms.

Identifying Personal Digital Triggers and Areas for Improvement

Each person's relationship with technology is unique, and so are the triggers that lead to excessive or unhealthy tech use. For some, it might be social media notifications; for others, the compulsion to check work emails after hours. Identifying your personal digital triggers can help you target specific areas for improvement. Reflect on which activities leave you feeling stressed, distracted, or unsatisfied, and look for patterns in your behavior.

Establishing Boundaries for Technology Use

Establishing boundaries for technology use is a key aspect of digital detoxification. This might involve setting time limits for certain activities (e.g., no more than an hour of social media per day), designating device-free zones in your home (e.g., no devices in the bedroom), or setting aside specific times for offline activities (e.g., reading, exercise, or spending time with loved ones).

Using digital well-being tools and settings on your devices can assist with this. For example, most smartphones now offer features to track screen time, set app limits, and enable 'do not disturb' modes.

Incorporating Regular Digital Detoxes into Daily Routines

Regular digital detoxes can help you maintain a healthy balance between online and offline activities. You might choose to have short daily detoxes (e.g., no devices for the first hour after waking and the hour before bed), weekly detoxes (e.g., a device-free day each weekend), or longer detoxes at intervals throughout the year.

Incorporating regular digital detoxes into your routine can provide opportunities to engage more deeply with offline activities and relationships, improve focus and productivity, and support overall well-being.

Remember, digital detoxification is not about completely rejecting technology, but about developing a healthier, more conscious relationship with it. By regularly stepping back from our devices, we can gain perspective, recharge, and return to our digital lives with a renewed sense of balance and control.

Balancing Digital and Offline Experiences

Balancing Digital and Offline Experiences

In the digital age, finding the right balance between our online and offline experiences is a challenge that requires continuous effort and mindfulness.

Strategies for Maintaining Balance and Mindfulness Post-Detox

1. Mindful Technology Use: Practicing mindful technology use involves being fully present and intentional with each digital interaction. It means asking yourself questions like, "Why am I picking up my device? Is this contributing positively to my life?" This awareness can help reduce unnecessary digital consumption.

2. Digital Sabbaticals: Regularly scheduled breaks from digital devices, or 'digital sabbaticals', can be an effective way to reset and regain perspective on our digital habits. These could range from a few hours each day to a weekend each month, or even a week-long break every few months.

3. Prioritizing Offline Activities: Make a list of activities you enjoy that don't involve digital devices, such as reading, hiking, painting, or playing a musical instrument. Prioritize these activities in your daily routine to ensure you have a healthy balance of offline experiences.

4. Quality over Quantity: Strive for quality rather than quantity in your digital interactions. Spend time on activities that add value to your life, and avoid mindless scrolling or excessive multi-tasking.

Incorporating Digital Minimalism Principles in Daily Life

1. Intentionality: Digital minimalism emphasizes intentional and deliberate use of technology. Before logging on to a device, define your purpose and stick to it. For example, if you're checking email, resist the urge to switch to social media.

2. Simplify: Regularly review and declutter your digital spaces. Unsubscribe from unnecessary emails, delete redundant apps, and tidy your virtual desktops. This simplification reduces digital distractions and makes technology use more efficiently and enjoyable.

3. Boundaries: Establish and maintain digital boundaries. These might include device-free times or zones, set hours for checking email or social media, or using technology-free methods for tasks like note-taking or reading.

4. Quality Interactions: Use technology to enhance your life, not detract from it. Focus on activities and interactions that add value, such as learning a new skill, connecting with loved ones, or contributing to your community.

By incorporating these strategies into daily life, you can cultivate a balanced and mindful approach to technology use that aligns with the principles of digital minimalism. Remember, the goal is not to eliminate digital technology, but to harness its benefits while minimizing its potential downsides.

The Importance of Nurturing Offline Relationships and Connections

While digital technology allows us to stay connected with people from around the world, it's essential not to neglect our offline relationships. Interacting face-to-face allows us to express and understand non-verbal cues, enhancing empathy and intimacy in our relationships. Offline interactions also provide a respite from screen time and offer a more authentic connection that cannot be replicated through a device.

Making time for offline interactions, such as regular family meals, catch-ups with friends, or community involvement, is crucial. These connections nourish our social wellbeing and remind us of our shared humanity, providing comfort, support, and a sense of belonging.

Engaging in Offline Hobbies and Activities for Relaxation and Personal Growth

Offline hobbies and activities play a vital role in relaxation, self-expression, and personal growth. They allow us to disconnect from the digital world, providing a break for our eyes and minds from screen time. These activities also offer opportunities to explore our interests, develop new skills, and express our creativity.

Whether it's painting, cooking, gardening, or playing a musical instrument, offline hobbies offer a form of active leisure that is more rewarding and fulfilling than passive screen time. They engage our minds in a different way, often providing a sense of achievement and progress that boosts our self-esteem and wellbeing.

The Role of Physical Exercise and Outdoor Activities in Promoting Overall Well-being

Physical exercise and outdoor activities offer significant benefits for our physical and mental health. Regular physical activity helps to maintain a healthy weight, reduce the risk of chronic diseases, and promote better sleep – all crucial for overall well-being. Furthermore, exercising outdoors provides additional benefits, including exposure to natural light, which aids our circadian rhythm and vitamin D synthesis.

Activities such as walking, cycling, hiking, or simply spending time in nature can help us disconnect from the digital world and reconnect with our surroundings. This reconnection can provide a sense of peace and perspective, reducing stress and promoting mental well-being.

Moreover, engaging in group sports or outdoor activities also presents opportunities to strengthen our offline social connections, providing a shared sense of camaraderie and belonging.

Balancing digital and offline experiences doesn't mean we should reject technology outright. Instead, it encourages us to use technology in a way that aligns with our life goals and values, fostering a healthier and more mindful relationship with our digital devices.

Building Long-term Habits for Digital Minimalism and Detoxification

Developing a Sustainable Approach to Digital Minimalism and Detoxification

Adopting digital minimalism and detoxification as long-term practices requires a sustainable approach. This approach involves not just a temporary break from digital devices but a fundamental shift in how we engage with technology. It requires setting personal rules that align with our values, priorities, and lifestyle.

A sustainable approach to digital minimalism may include strategies such as setting specific times for checking emails or social media, turning off non-essential notifications, or using technology tools that help limit screen time. It's not about completely eliminating digital devices from our lives, but using them in a way that serves us without causing stress or distraction.

Practicing digital detox regularly is also essential for a sustainable approach. This could be as simple as designating certain times of the day as device-free, or setting aside a full day each week where you disconnect entirely from digital devices. Over time, these regular breaks can help recalibrate our relationship with technology, making it easier to maintain minimalistic practices.

Overcoming Challenges and Setbacks in Maintaining Digital Minimalism Practices

Transitioning to digital minimalism can be challenging, particularly given our society's heavy reliance on technology. Setbacks are not only common but also a normal part of the process. What matters is how we respond to these challenges and continue to strive towards our goal of digital minimalism.

Firstly, it's important to remember why you decided to adopt digital minimalism. Whether it's to reduce anxiety, improve focus, or have more time for offline activities, reminding yourself of these reasons can provide motivation to continue when faced with challenges.

Secondly, try to identify the specific triggers or situations that lead to setbacks. For instance, if you find yourself mindlessly scrolling through social media when you're bored, consider other activities you could do instead, such as reading a book, going for a walk, or calling a friend.

Lastly, be patient with yourself. Changing habits takes time, and it's okay to have moments of relapse. What's important is to acknowledge the setback, learn from it, and then get back on track. Celebrate your progress, no matter how small, and remember that the journey to digital minimalism is a marathon, not a sprint. It's about making small, incremental changes that, over time, lead to a healthier relationship with digital technology.

Fostering a Supportive Network and Community for Embracing Digital Minimalism

To sustain digital minimalism in the long run, a supportive network is essential. This could be family, friends, or a broader community who understand and respect your goals. By sharing your objectives with your close ones, you invite them to support you in your journey. They can provide motivation during challenging times and celebrate your milestones with you.

Additionally, seek out communities of digital minimalists, both online and offline. These communities can offer encouragement, share personal experiences, and provide practical advice. They can also help normalize digital minimalism, making it easier to resist societal pressures to always be connected.

Practical Steps for Implementing Digital Minimalism and Detoxification

There are several practical steps you can take to implement and maintain digital minimalism and detoxification:

1. Declutter Your Digital Environment: Start by simplifying your digital spaces. This could involve unsubscribing from unnecessary emails, deleting unused apps, or clearing out old files and documents. Like a clean physical workspace, a decluttered digital environment can increase focus and reduce stress.

2. Set Boundaries for Digital Usage: Define clear boundaries for when and how you use your digital devices. This could mean setting specific times for checking emails or social media, creating device-free zones in your home, or turning off notifications during certain hours.

3. Tips for a Successful Digital Detox: Start small, such as by setting aside a few hours each day without digital devices. As you become more comfortable, you can gradually increase the length of your detox. During this time, engage in activities that you enjoy and that help you relax, such as reading, walking, or meditating. Remember to inform your close ones about your detox plans, so they can provide support and not worry if they can't reach you during those times.

4. Regular Check-ins: Regularly assess your relationship with digital technology. Are you falling back into old habits? Are there new challenges you need to address? Regular check-ins can help you stay on track and make necessary adjustments.

5. Patience and Persistence: Changing habits takes time. Be patient with yourself and remember that it's okay to have setbacks. What's important is to persist. Each step, no matter how small, brings you closer to a healthier relationship with digital technology.

Digital minimalism is not about completely abandoning digital devices, but about using them in a more intentional and balanced way. By adopting these strategies, you can create a digital lifestyle that aligns with your personal values and enhances your overall well-being.

Mindful Technology Use and Healthy Habits

Understanding Mindful Technology Use

Understanding Mindful Technology Use

In the digital age, technology has permeated every aspect of our lives. The ubiquity of digital devices has led to an 'always-on' culture, where we are constantly connected and continually consuming information. While there are many benefits to this digital connectivity, it can also lead to stress, anxiety, and a sense of being overwhelmed. This is where the concept of mindful technology use comes in.

Mindful technology use refers to the conscious, intentional use of technology. It involves being fully present and aware of how we are using our devices, rather than using them on autopilot. It means consciously choosing to engage with technology in ways that are beneficial and productive, rather than letting it dictate our actions and reactions.

The Concept of Mindfulness in the Context of Technology Use

Mindfulness, at its core, is about being fully present and engaged in the current moment. It involves focusing our attention on what we are doing, thinking, or feeling right now, without judgment or distraction. In the context of technology use, mindfulness translates to being fully aware of our digital actions and their impacts on our well-being.

For example, are we reaching for our phone out of habit or necessity? Are we mindlessly scrolling through social media, or are we intentionally seeking out information or connection? Are we using technology to avoid negative feelings or to genuinely enhance our lives?

The Benefits of Mindful Technology Use for Mental Health and Well-being

1. Reduced Stress and Anxiety: By using technology mindfully, we can reduce the feelings of stress and anxiety associated with constant connectivity and information overload. We can choose to engage with digital content that uplifts us rather than drains us, and we can take breaks when needed without feeling guilty or anxious.

2. Improved Focus and Productivity: When we use technology with intention, we can minimize distractions and improve our focus. This can lead to greater productivity and a sense of accomplishment.

3. Better Sleep: Mindful technology use can improve our sleep by reducing our exposure to screens before bedtime and by minimizing the stress and anxiety that can interfere with a good night's sleep.

4. Enhanced Relationships: By being fully present in our interactions with others, both online and offline, we can build stronger, more meaningful relationships.

5. Greater Self-Awareness and Self-Control: Mindful technology use can increase our self-awareness of our digital habits and their impacts on our well-being. This awareness can lead to greater self-control and the ability to make healthier digital choices.

Mindful technology use is about using technology as a tool to enhance our lives, rather than letting it control us. By bringing mindfulness to our digital interactions, we can promote healthier digital habits, improve our mental health, and enhance our overall well-being.

Techniques for Cultivating Mindful Technology Use

Techniques for Cultivating Mindful Technology Use

In the digital era where technology is deeply integrated into our lives, cultivating mindful technology use can seem daunting. However, it is achievable with the application of various techniques that blend mindfulness principles with our daily interactions with technology.

Mindfulness Exercises and Practices for Technology Use

1. Mindful Notifications: Notifications have become one of the major sources of digital distraction. The first step towards mindful technology use involves being intentional about which applications can send notifications. Limiting notifications to essential apps can reduce digital noise and help us stay focused on our current tasks.

2. Mindful Scrolling: Mindless scrolling is a common habit that can lead to wasted time and a sense of digital overload. A mindful scrolling exercise involves setting a purpose for each digital session. Before opening an app, we can ask ourselves, "What is my intention for using this app right now?" This can help us stay focused and prevent us from falling into the scrolling trap.

3. Mindful Emailing: Emails can often become a source of stress, especially when our inbox is overflowing. A mindful emailing practice involves setting specific times for checking and responding to emails rather than constantly checking throughout the day. It also involves being mindful of the tone and content of our emails, ensuring they are clear, concise, and respectful.

4. Digital Mindfulness Meditation: This involves taking short breaks during the day to do a quick mindfulness meditation. This could be as simple as closing our eyes and focusing on our breath for a few minutes. There are also numerous apps available that offer guided digital mindfulness meditations.

The Role of Regular Self-Reflection and Assessment in Promoting Mindful Technology Use

Regular self-reflection and assessment play a crucial role in promoting mindful technology use. By taking time to reflect on our digital habits, we can gain a deeper understanding of our relationship with technology and identify areas for improvement.

1. Digital Use Journaling: Keeping a journal of our daily technology use can provide valuable insights into our digital habits. We can record when we use technology, what we use it for, and how it makes us feel. Over time, patterns may emerge that highlight our digital triggers and habits.

2. Digital Self-Assessment: Regularly evaluating our digital health can help us stay mindful of our technology use. This might involve asking ourselves questions like: "Am I spending too much time on certain apps?"; "Is my technology use interfering with my sleep or productivity?"; "Am I using technology to avoid certain feelings or situations?"

3. Mindful Goal Setting: Based on our self-reflection and assessment, we can set mindful technology use goals. These goals should be specific, measurable, achievable, relevant, and time-bound (SMART). For example, we might set a goal to limit our social media use to 30 minutes per day or to not check email after 8 pm.

4. Regular Digital Detoxes: Regular digital detoxes, where we intentionally disconnect from technology for a certain period, can be a powerful way to reset our digital habits and cultivate mindful technology use. This could be as short as an hour each day, a day each week, or a week each year – whatever feels achievable and beneficial.

Mindful technology use is not about completely eliminating technology from our lives, but about using it in a way that serves us rather than controls us. By incorporating mindfulness exercises into our technology use and regularly reflecting on our digital habits, we can cultivate a healthier relationship with our devices and improve our overall digital wellbeing.

Strategies for Setting and Maintaining Boundaries with Digital Devices

In a world where digital devices are deeply interwoven into our lives, setting boundaries with technology is vital. It's about striking a balance between harnessing the benefits of technology and avoiding its potential drawbacks. We will explore the strategies for setting and maintaining boundaries with digital devices and provide insights on navigating the challenges and obstacles in boundary-setting.

1. Time-Based Boundaries: One of the most effective strategies for setting boundaries with technology is to create time-based rules. This could involve setting specific hours for work-related technology use, scheduling time for digital leisure activities, or establishing a digital curfew, a specific time in the evening after which you avoid all digital devices to ensure a good night's sleep.

2. Space-Based Boundaries: Allocating specific areas in your home for technology use can be another useful strategy. This could involve designating a specific workstation for work-related tasks, setting a rule of no devices at the dinner table or creating a device-free zone in the bedroom to promote better sleep.

3. Activity-Based Boundaries: Limiting technology use during certain activities can also be an effective way of setting boundaries. For instance, you might decide to avoid digital devices when spending time with loved ones, exercising, or engaging in hobbies. This can enhance the quality of these activities and help to foster stronger real-life connections.

4. Digital Wellbeing Tools: Many digital devices and applications now come with built-in features that can help you monitor and manage your technology use. This can be a helpful aid in setting and maintaining boundaries, as these tools can provide insights into your usage patterns and help you set limits on your device use.

5. Mindfulness Practices: Incorporating mindfulness practices into your technology use can also assist in setting boundaries. By being fully present and intentional when using digital devices, you can avoid mindless scrolling and ensure your technology use aligns with your personal values and goals.

Navigating Challenges and Obstacles in Boundary-Setting

Setting boundaries with technology is not without its challenges. However, understanding these obstacles can help in navigating them effectively.

1. Fear of Missing Out (FOMO): This is a common challenge when setting boundaries with technology. We often worry about missing out on important updates or being left out of social interactions. However, it's essential to remember that real-life connections and personal wellbeing should take precedence over digital interactions. Remind yourself of the benefits of setting boundaries and the value of quality over quantity when it comes to digital engagement.

2. Work Demands: In today's digital work culture, setting boundaries can often be difficult due to expectations of constant availability. It's important to communicate your boundaries clearly to your colleagues and superiors and to advocate for a healthy work-life balance.

3. Habitual Behavior: Technology use can often become a habitual behavior or a reflexive action. Breaking these habits can be challenging, but mindful technology use, self-reflection, and gradual changes can help in overcoming this obstacle.

4. External Pressure: Sometimes, the pressure to engage in digital activities comes from friends, family, or societal norms. It's important to stand firm in your boundaries and explain to others why these boundaries are important to you.

5. Digital Detox: Occasionally, taking a break from technology can be a good way to reset your digital habits. However, these detoxes should be planned carefully to avoid feeling overwhelmed when you reintegrate technology back into your life.

Setting boundaries with technology is a personal journey that will look different for everyone. It's about finding a balance that allows you to enjoy the benefits of technology without compromising your mental health and well-being. By understanding the strategies for setting boundaries and the potential challenges

Building Healthy Digital Habits

As we navigate through an era where digital technology is an integral part of our lives, building healthy digital habits is crucial. The right habits can enhance our productivity, improve our mental health, and foster better relationships. See some useful tips for developing and reinforcing healthy digital habits, discussing the importance of consistency and self-compassion in habit formation, and highlighting ways to cultivate a supportive environment for mindful technology use.

Tips for Developing and Reinforcing Healthy Digital Habits

1. Start Small: When developing a new habit, it's important to start small. Focus on one habit at a time, and break it down into manageable steps. For instance, if your goal is to reduce social media consumption, start by setting a limit on one platform before tackling others.

2. Be Specific: Specificity can help reinforce habits. Rather than setting a vague goal like "spend less time on my phone," set a concrete goal like "use my phone for no more than two hours a day."

3. Prioritize High-Value Activities: Make a list of activities that provide real value - whether that's professional development, relaxation, or connection with others. Prioritize these activities over mindless scrolling or excessive digital consumption.

4. Use Tools to Help: Many digital devices come with built-in tools that can help you manage your screen time, set reminders for breaks, or block certain applications during specific times. Use these to your advantage.

5. Establish Routine Checks: Regularly review your digital habits to see if they align with your goals. Self-reflection can help identify areas of improvement and reinforce positive behaviors.

The Role of Consistency and Self-Compassion in Habit Formation

1. Consistency: Consistency is key in habit formation. It's better to engage in a small, new behavior consistently than to attempt a major change all at once and not be able to sustain it. Over time, consistent actions become automatic, leading to long-lasting habits.

2. Self-Compassion: Building new habits is a process, and there will be setbacks. It's essential to practice self-compassion during this process. Don't be too hard on yourself if you deviate from your goals; instead, recognize the misstep and use it as a learning experience to guide future actions.

Cultivating a Supportive Environment for Mindful Technology Use

1. Digital Spaces: Tailor your digital spaces to support your new habits. This could involve decluttering your digital environment, customizing your notifications, or curating your online feeds to align with your goals.

2. Physical Spaces: Your physical environment can also influence your digital habits. Designate specific areas for technology use and device-free zones to encourage mindful technology use.

3. Social Support: Inform your friends, family, or colleagues about your new digital habits. Their understanding and support can make the transition smoother. Plus, you might inspire them to adopt healthier digital habits too!

4. Professional Help: If you find it challenging to change your digital habits, don't hesitate to seek professional help. Therapists, counselors, and life coaches can provide valuable guidance and resources.

Building healthy digital habits is a journey that requires commitment, patience, and effort. However, with the right strategies, consistent effort, self-compassion, and a supportive environment, we can all cultivate digital habits that improve our lives and well-being in the digital age.

Leveraging Technology for Mental Health Support

The Advent of Online Therapy

In the digital age, where technology has permeated every facet of our lives, it has also transformed how we approach mental health. The advent of online therapy has made it easier for people to access support and manage their mental health, breaking down barriers such as stigma, location, and time. We will explore the concept and benefits of online therapy and see guidance on choosing an online therapy platform that aligns with individual needs.

Understanding the Concept and Benefits of Online Therapy

Online therapy, also known as teletherapy or e-therapy, involves providing mental health services over the internet. These services can be offered through various mediums such as video conferencing, phone calls, text messaging, or mobile apps. This digital approach to therapy has revolutionized mental health care, making it more accessible and convenient.

1. Accessibility: Online therapy has made mental health services more accessible. It eliminates geographic barriers, making it easier for people in remote or underserved areas to access quality mental health care. It also provides a solution for those who may have mobility challenges or hectic schedules.

2. Convenience: The convenience of online therapy cannot be understated. Appointments can be scheduled at a time that suits the client's schedule, and therapy sessions can take place in the comfort of one's home.

3. Anonymity: For some people, the perceived stigma associated with seeking mental health support can be a deterrent. Online therapy offers a level of anonymity that can make it easier for us to seek help.

4. Cost-effectiveness: In many cases, online therapy can be more cost-effective than traditional in-person therapy, making mental health support more affordable.

How to Choose an Online Therapy Platform That Suits Your Needs

With a myriad of online therapy platforms available, it can be challenging to choose the right one. Here are some factors to consider when making your decision:

1. Credibility: The most important factor is the credibility of the platform. Ensure that the therapists are licensed professionals and that the platform adheres to strict privacy and confidentiality guidelines. Look for reviews and testimonials to gauge the effectiveness of the therapy provided.

2. Therapeutic Approach: Different therapists use different therapeutic approaches. Some may use cognitive-behavioral therapy (CBT), while others may use dialectical behavior therapy (DBT) or other modalities. Ensure that the platform you choose offers the therapeutic approach that aligns with your needs and preferences.

3. Cost: Online therapy platforms vary in cost. Some offer a subscription model, while others charge per session. Consider your budget and the cost-effectiveness of the platform. Some platforms may also offer financial aid or sliding scale fees.

4. User Experience: Consider the user experience of the platform. Is it easy to navigate? Does it offer features that enhance the therapeutic experience, such as journaling tools, mindfulness exercises, or mood tracking?

5. Specializations: If you're seeking help for a specific issue, such as anxiety, depression, PTSD, or relationship issues, look for a platform that offers therapists who specialize in that area.

The advent of online therapy has ushered in a new era of mental health support, making therapy more accessible, convenient, and cost-effective. However, it's crucial to choose an online therapy platform that suits your individual needs and preferences, to get the most out of the experience. As we continue to leverage technology for mental health support, we move closer to a world where everyone has access to the mental health care they need.

Mental Health Apps: A Handy Support

In the realm of mental health support, the digital landscape is flourishing with resources. One of the most significant developments has been the advent of mental health applications. These apps, available at the touch of a screen, are designed to provide a range of services from mood tracking and meditation to therapy and peer support.

The beauty of this digital revolution in mental health care is the vast array of options available. Each application comes with its unique set of features, tailored to address different aspects of mental health. This diversity caters to the individuality of our mental health journeys, acknowledging that what works for one person may not work for another. As such, the power lies in your hands to explore and decide which resources align with your needs and preferences.

We will explore a range of mental health apps, examining their unique features to provide you with a comprehensive overview. Remember, these are just a few examples in a sea of possibilities. The aim here is not to prescribe a 'one-size-fits-all' solution, but to equip you with knowledge about what's available, so you can make an informed choice about what tools to incorporate into your mental health toolkit.

Remember, while these apps offer valuable support, they are not a replacement for professional help, especially in situations requiring immediate attention or in cases of severe mental health conditions.

Exploration of Various Mental Health Apps and Their Features

Exploration of Various Mental Health Apps and Their Features
In the digital era, mental health support has expanded beyond traditional face-to-face therapy. A plethora of mental health applications are now available at our fingertips, providing a range of services to cater to diverse needs.

Mood-Tracking Apps:

Mood-tracking apps are designed to allow us to log and monitor our emotional states over time. A prime example is Moodpath, an interactive mental health screening and improvement app. It asks users daily questions to assess their well-being and provides bi-weekly mental health assessments. It can generate an electronic document summarizing the user's mood over a specified period, which can be shared with a healthcare professional.

Daylio is another mood-tracking app that allows users to keep a private journal without having to type a single line. Users pick their mood and add activities they have been doing during the day. Over time, this app can help users discover patterns and habits associated with different moods.

Mindfulness and Meditation Apps:

Applications such as Headspace and Calm promote mindfulness and meditation. Headspace provides guided meditations, animations, articles, and videos in a fun and friendly approach. It offers a variety of courses on topics ranging from managing stress and anxiety to promoting healthier sleep.

Calm, on the other hand, is renowned for its sleep stories – bedtime stories for adults designed to aid in a peaceful night's sleep. It also offers meditation programs, relaxing music, and nature sounds.

Therapy Apps:

Therapy apps connect users with licensed therapists for digital therapy sessions. Talkspace offers users the ability to text, voice message, or live video call with their allocated licensed therapist. It covers a broad range of therapy types, including individual therapy, couples therapy, and adolescent therapy.

Another similar platform is BetterHelp, which matches users to licensed therapists based on a questionnaire. Users can communicate via messaging, live chat, phone, and video sessions.

Self-Help Apps:

Self-help apps offer strategies based on various mental health therapies. Happify uses games and activities based on cognitive-behavioral therapy, positive psychology, and mindfulness to help users overcome stress, anxiety, and negative thoughts.

Sanvello is designed to help users manage symptoms of stress, anxiety, and depression. It offers daily mood tracking, guided journeys, coping tools, and a community board for peer support.

Peer Support Apps:

Peer support apps provide a platform for users to connect with others experiencing similar mental health concerns. Wisdo connects users based on shared experiences, providing a platform to learn from others who have been in the same situation.

7 Cups offers free emotional support from trained volunteer listeners, alongside paid therapy options. The platform also includes community forums for more general peer support.

Exploring these various mental health apps can assist us in identifying resources that suit our specific needs and preferences. Each app has distinct features and focuses, providing a diverse range of options for users seeking digital mental health support. Remember, while these apps can be beneficial, they should not replace professional help, especially in severe or crisis situations.

Maximizing the Benefits of Mental Health Apps

To maximize the benefits of mental health apps, it's essential to use them effectively and safely:

1. Choose Wisely: Given the multitude of mental health apps available, selecting one that suits your needs is crucial. Review the app's features, user reviews, and privacy policies. It's also beneficial if the app's content is developed or reviewed by licensed mental health professionals.

2. Consistency is Key: Like any mental health intervention, consistency is key when using these apps. Regular use increases the likelihood of improvement in mental health symptoms.

3. Complement, Not Replace: Mental health apps should be viewed as a complement to traditional mental health treatments rather than a replacement. They are an excellent tool for managing symptoms and practicing self-care but should not replace professional help, especially in severe cases.

4. Engage with Features: Many mental health apps provide a variety of features, such as mood tracking, mindfulness exercises, and cognitive-behavioral therapy activities. Regularly engaging with these features can maximize the app's benefits.

5. Maintain Privacy: Ensure that the app has stringent privacy policies in place. As you may be sharing sensitive information, it's essential to choose an app that respects and protects your data.

Mental health apps can be a valuable tool for supporting mental health and well-being. They offer a range of services, from mood tracking and mindfulness exercises to therapy sessions and peer support, right at our fingertips. While they don't replace professional help, they can certainly complement traditional therapy, offering accessible and convenient resources to manage mental health on a daily basis. By understanding their features and using them effectively, we can leverage these digital tools to support our mental health journey.

Virtual Support Groups: Finding Community Online

In our journey towards improved mental health, we are not alone. The digital age has brought forth an array of platforms that create opportunities for us to connect with others who share similar experiences, feelings, and struggles. Virtual support groups are one such offering, becoming an increasingly important resource for many of us navigating mental health challenges. They provide an accessible, convenient, and often less intimidating alternative to face-to-face meetings, thus breaking down barriers to help-seeking behavior and enabling us to find solace in community online.

The Role and Importance of Virtual Support Groups

Virtual support groups play an integral role in our mental health journeys. They serve as a safe space where we can share our experiences, learn from others, and feel a sense of belonging. This is particularly crucial for those of us who might feel isolated or misunderstood in our day-to-day lives due to our mental health challenges.

These online communities provide an opportunity to connect with others who understand what we're going through. They help normalize our feelings and experiences, reducing feelings of isolation. We can benefit from the collective wisdom of others who have walked the path before us, gaining insights into coping strategies, resources, and therapies that have proven effective.

In addition, the anonymity that online platforms provide can make it easier for us to open up about our struggles without the fear of judgment or stigma. This can be particularly valuable for those of us dealing with highly stigmatized conditions or those of us who may not feel comfortable discussing our mental health concerns in our immediate social circles.

How to Participate and Gain Support in Online Mental Health Communities

Participating in virtual support groups can be an empowering and enlightening experience, but it's important to approach them with an open mind and respect for the shared space. Firstly, it's crucial to remember that each of us is at a different point in our journey, and the pace of progress may vary greatly. Patience, empathy, and understanding should be the guiding principles of our interactions within these groups.

When participating in these groups, it's okay to start as a silent observer. Reading others' experiences and seeing how they are supported can help us feel more comfortable and understand the dynamics of the group. As we grow more comfortable, we can begin to share our experiences, thoughts, and feelings at our own pace. It's important to remember that there's no pressure to share until we feel ready.

When sharing, we should strive to be honest yet considerate. It's crucial to be aware that while it's a safe space to express ourselves, our words can impact others. We should avoid offering direct advice unless asked, as what worked for us might not necessarily work for others.

Finally, it's important to remember that while virtual support groups are a valuable resource, they don't replace professional mental health treatment. They should be used as a supplementary support system. If we find ourselves in a crisis or in need of professional help, we should reach out to a mental health professional directly.

Finding our community online can be an essential step towards feeling less alone in our mental health journey. Virtual support groups provide a space where we can find understanding, acceptance, and mutual support. With respect and empathy as our guide, we can both offer and receive support in these digital spaces, enhancing our overall well-being.

Telemedicine and Mental Health

As we traverse the digital age, telemedicine has emerged as a transformative tool, reshaping the way we access and receive mental health care. This technology-driven approach to healthcare has been on the rise, especially in the field of mental health. Its potential to bridge gaps in access to care, provide convenience, and offer personalized support is unparalleled. However, like any other innovation, telemedicine also presents its unique set of challenges.

The Rise of Telemedicine in Mental Health Care

Telemedicine, a practice that involves providing medical services remotely via digital platforms, has seen a significant surge in recent years. This rise can be attributed to several factors. For one, our digital proficiency has increased, making us more comfortable with using online platforms for various needs, including healthcare. Additionally, the need for remote healthcare solutions has been amplified by global crises like the COVID-19 pandemic, which limited in-person interactions.

In the realm of mental health, the rise of telemedicine has been particularly notable. The nature of mental health services, often centered around talking therapies, makes them highly suitable for delivery via digital means. We can engage in therapeutic conversations, receive guidance and support, and progress in our mental health journeys without the need for physical proximity to a healthcare provider.

Benefits of Telemedicine for Mental Health Support

Telemedicine offers numerous benefits for mental health support. Firstly, it improves access to mental health services, especially for us in remote areas or those with limited mobility. It breaks down geographical barriers, allowing us to receive care from the comfort of our own homes.

Telemedicine also affords us the luxury of flexibility. We can schedule appointments at times that suit us, saving time and reducing stress associated with travel. It can make therapy more appealing and less daunting, especially for those of us who might feel anxious about in-person sessions.

Additionally, telemedicine can provide a sense of anonymity that some of us might find comforting. It can help alleviate concerns about stigma associated with seeking mental health support, encouraging us to take the crucial step towards getting help.

Challenges of Telemedicine for Mental Health Support

Despite its numerous advantages, telemedicine is not without its challenges. One significant issue is the digital divide. Not all of us have access to stable internet connections or digital devices needed for telemedicine, which can widen existing disparities in mental health care.

Another concern is that of privacy and security. Confidentiality is fundamental to mental health services, and digital platforms can be susceptible to data breaches. Therefore, it's crucial for telemedicine providers to prioritize robust security measures to protect our information.

Also, while telemedicine can be incredibly convenient, it may not be suitable for all types of mental health interventions. Some therapeutic techniques require in-person interaction. Furthermore, the absence of physical cues might make it challenging for healthcare providers to fully grasp our emotional state.

Lastly, building a therapeutic alliance, which is key to successful therapy outcomes, might be more challenging in a virtual setting. Some of us might find it more difficult to connect with our therapists over a screen.

The rise of telemedicine in mental health care has the potential to reshape our approach to mental health support, making it more accessible and convenient. However, it's important to navigate its challenges mindfully to ensure we receive the best care possible. As we continue to evolve with the digital age, we can hope for a future where these challenges are addressed, making telemedicine a robust and inclusive solution for mental health care.

Navigating Digital Mental Health Resources Responsibly

As the use of digital mental health resources continues to grow, it is imperative that we equip ourselves with the knowledge and skills needed to navigate these tools responsibly. These resources offer a wide array of benefits, but they also come with certain challenges that we must be prepared to handle effectively. Moreover, while these digital tools are valuable, it's crucial to strike a balance between digital and traditional mental health support to ensure our overall well-being.

Guidelines for Using Digital Mental Health Resources Responsibly and Effectively

Using digital mental health resources requires a responsible approach to ensure they serve our needs effectively. Here are some guidelines to help us navigate this journey:

1. Research and verify: Before using any digital mental health tool, we need to conduct thorough research. Look for reviews, check the credibility of the source, and ensure it's a recognized and trustworthy platform. Ensure the information provided aligns with scientific understanding and is backed by mental health professionals.

2. Privacy and security: Digital platforms pose potential risks to our privacy. Therefore, we should be vigilant about the security measures in place on these platforms. Check the privacy policy and data handling practices before sharing any personal information.

3. Avoid self-diagnosis: While digital resources can provide valuable information and support, they should not replace professional diagnosis or treatment. If we are experiencing mental health difficulties, it is crucial to seek professional help.

4. Maintain realistic expectations: Digital mental health resources can provide support and aid in our mental health journey, but they are not a magic solution. We need to be patient, consistent, and realistic about what these tools can offer.

Strategies for Maintaining a Balance Between Digital and Traditional Mental Health Support

While digital resources provide accessibility and convenience, traditional mental health support remains an integral part of our mental health care. Here are some strategies to maintain a healthy balance:

1. Supplement, not replace: We should view digital resources as a supplement to traditional mental health support, not a replacement. In-person therapy, group support, and medication (if prescribed) are essential components of many mental health treatment plans.

2. Face-to-face connections: Human connection plays a vital role in our mental health. Engaging in face-to-face interactions with our loved ones, community members, or mental health professionals is crucial, even as we leverage digital resources.

3. Digital Detox: Regularly disconnecting from digital devices can help maintain our mental health. Scheduling device-free time or days can provide necessary respite and help us stay connected to our real-world experiences.

4. Mindful usage: Be mindful of the time spent using digital mental health resources. Set boundaries to ensure we are not over-relying on these tools at the expense of other important aspects of our lives.

Navigating digital mental health resources responsibly is an important skill in our digital age. By following the guidelines for responsible use and maintaining a balance between digital and traditional mental health support, we can make the most of these resources while preserving our overall well-being. The journey might seem challenging, but with a mindful and informed approach, we can effectively leverage these tools to bolster our mental health journey.

Navigating The Digital Age with Intention and Balance

Reflecting on the Digital Landscape

In the digital era, where our lives are intertwined with technology more than ever, understanding and navigating the digital landscape becomes crucial for our overall well-being. This journey through the digital landscape has shed light on various facets of our digital lives, ranging from cyberbullying to digital minimalism, from mindful technology use to leveraging technology for mental health support.

Cyberbullying and online harassment emerged as pressing issues in our digital society. We have learned to identify different forms of cyberbullying, the psychological effects they inflict, and the role of social media platforms in either facilitating or mitigating such harm. The importance of digital literacy and education in preventing such occurrences were underscored. Strategies were outlined to help us recognize, report, and cope with cyberbullying and online harassment, highlighting the need for empathy, kindness, and positive digital citizenship in the online environment.

In response to these online challenges, we dived into the importance of digital resilience, focusing on emotional, cognitive, and behavioral resilience. This holistic approach to resilience equips us to recognize and manage emotions tied to online experiences, engage in critical thinking when consuming online information, and cultivate healthy digital habits. Through the lens of resilience, we learned that it's not just about 'surviving' the digital age, but indeed 'thriving' within it.

Digital minimalism and detoxification were highlighted as essential practices for managing our digital consumption. The principles of digital minimalism were explored, and various strategies for digital detoxification were provided. The focus was not only on reducing digital use but also on intentional and mindful engagement with digital content.

Mindful technology use emerged as a significant theme in our journey. We explored techniques for cultivating mindfulness in our interactions with technology, setting boundaries, and building healthy digital habits. This mindfulness-based approach to technology use is a potent antidote to digital overload and distraction, bringing intentionality and balance into our digital lives.

The latter part of our exploration brought to light the possibilities of leveraging technology for mental health support. The advent of online therapy, mental health apps, virtual support groups, and telemedicine were discussed as potential resources that can complement traditional mental health support systems. Guidelines for using these resources responsibly and effectively were provided, underscoring the need for balance between digital and traditional mental health support.

Navigating the digital landscape with intention and balance is a skill that needs cultivation. It's about being proactive in our digital lives, making conscious choices about our digital consumption, and leveraging the positive aspects of technology for our well-being. The insights gleaned from this journey equip us not just to survive, but thrive, in the digital age.

As we continue our journey in the digital age, it's essential to remember that technology is a tool. And like any tool, its impact on our lives depends largely on how we use it. Let's use it with intention, mindfulness, and a spirit of digital resilience, creating a digital world that supports our well-being and growth.

The Balance Between Offline and Online

Striking the Right Balance

Striking the right balance between online and offline experiences is crucial in today's digital age. Our journey thus far has underscored the importance of maintaining a healthy balance between our digital and non-digital activities.

Understanding the impact of the digital world on our lives is the first step in achieving this balance. The digital environment provides us with a vast array of resources, opportunities, and platforms for connection. However, overindulgence or misuse of these platforms can lead to a range of challenges, from mental health issues such as anxiety and depression, to reduced productivity and disrupted relationships. By recognizing these potential issues, we can create a more mindful approach to our digital engagement, one that prioritizes our well-being.

The principles of digital minimalism and detoxification emerged as powerful strategies for achieving this balance. As we explored, these approaches encourage us to declutter our digital lives, be more intentional with our technology use, and engage in regular digital detoxes. The goal is not to eliminate digital technology from our lives, but to use it in a way that adds value and meaning, rather than detracting from our well-being.

Offline experiences, as we discovered, play a vital role in this balance. Engaging in offline hobbies, nurturing our offline relationships, and spending time in nature are not just enjoyable activities; they are essential for our physical and mental health. They provide a counterbalance to our digital experiences, ensuring that our lives are rich and varied.

Physical exercise and outdoor activities, in particular, emerged as crucial elements in balancing our digital and non-digital lives. These activities help to alleviate the physical and mental strains associated with excessive screen time, promote better sleep, and enhance our overall well-being.

In terms of practical steps to achieve this balance, setting boundaries emerged as a key strategy. By establishing clear rules for our technology use, such as device-free zones and times, we can ensure that our digital activities do not encroach on our offline lives. Mindful technology use, as we explored, is not about strict rules or complete abstinence but about conscious, intentional engagement.

Consistency and self-compassion, as we've learned, are crucial in maintaining this balance. Striving for perfection or drastic changes can often lead to frustration and failure. Instead, it's about making small, consistent changes, and being kind to ourselves when we encounter setbacks.

Support networks play an essential role in our digital balance. Whether it's family, friends, or online communities, these networks can provide encouragement, advice, and accountability, helping us to stay on track.

As we move forward, let's remember that achieving balance in our digital lives is not a destination, but a journey. It's a continuous process of learning, adapting, and making conscious choices. The strategies and insights we have gleaned from our journey equip us to navigate this balance with greater confidence and resilience.

The balance between our online and offline lives is not just a matter of time management; it's a question of how we want to live our lives. By making intentional choices, setting boundaries, and maintaining a strong connection with our offline world, we can create a digital life that supports our well-being and aligns with our values.

Intentional Use of Technology

Harnessing Technology with Purpose

In our exploration of the digital landscape, the concept of intentional technology use emerged as a fundamental principle. Intentional technology use involves engaging with digital devices and platforms purposefully, mindfully, and in ways that contribute positively to our lives. We will recap the main points we've covered on this topic and how we can apply this principle to our daily lives.

Understanding the concept of intentional technology use is the first step. It goes beyond mere functionality or convenience; it's about making conscious decisions about why, when, and how we use technology. It means asking ourselves if our digital activities align with our goals, values, and well-being, and making adjustments where necessary. This approach helps to prevent the misuse or overuse of technology, promoting a healthier, more balanced digital life.

The practice of intentional technology use requires regular self-reflection and assessment. We need to continually evaluate our digital habits and their impact on our lives. This might involve keeping a digital diary, setting aside time each week to reflect on our online activities, or even using digital wellness tools to track our screen time. Such reflection allows us to identify areas for improvement and make informed decisions about our digital behavior.

In terms of applying this concept to everyday life, several strategies came to the fore. Setting boundaries with technology emerged as a crucial step. This might involve creating device-free zones in our homes, setting specific times for checking emails or social media, or even scheduling regular digital detoxes. These boundaries help to ensure that technology serves us, rather than the other way around.

Digital minimalism was another significant strategy. This approach encourages us to declutter our digital lives, focusing on high-value activities that genuinely add to our lives, and discarding those that don't. By reducing digital noise and distractions, we can engage more meaningfully and productively with our online activities.

Mindfulness practices also play a key role in intentional technology use. As we explored, mindfulness can help us to engage more fully with our online activities, reducing mindless scrolling and promoting deeper, more satisfying digital experiences. Whether it's pausing before we check our phones, taking a few deep breaths before responding to an email, or simply paying full attention to a single online task, these practices can greatly enhance our digital well-being.

Moreover, we need to cultivate healthy digital habits, such as taking regular screen breaks, prioritizing offline connections, and ensuring we have a good digital posture. Consistency, patience, and self-compassion are crucial here; forming new habits takes time, and there will inevitably be setbacks along the way.

Finally, remember that intentional technology use is a personal journey. What works for one person might not work for another. It's about finding a digital balance that suits our unique needs, goals, and circumstances.

Intentional technology use is not about rejecting technology, but about harnessing its power in ways that enrich our lives. By engaging with technology mindfully, setting clear boundaries, and cultivating healthy digital habits, we can navigate the digital world with greater confidence and resilience. As we continue our digital journey, let's strive to make each click, swipe, and scroll a conscious, purposeful action.

Future Directions: The Evolving Digital Age

Navigating the Future of Our Digital World

As we journey deeper into the digital age, we must be prepared for continual evolution and change. Technology and its use will persist in shifting, and the landscape may look significantly different in the coming years.

In our exploration of the digital age, we have considered the profound impact technology has on our mental health. From the role of social media in shaping our self-perceptions and relationships to the effects of digital overload on our stress levels and productivity, it's clear that our digital behaviors profoundly influence our well-being. Looking ahead, these dynamics are likely to intensify as technology becomes more integrated into our daily lives.

Future trends in technology, such as artificial intelligence, virtual and augmented reality, and the continued rise of remote work and digital communication, have the potential to reshape our digital experiences. While these advances offer exciting opportunities for efficiency, connection, and entertainment, they also pose new challenges for our mental health.

For example, AI and machine learning could lead to more personalized and immersive digital experiences, but they could also increase our screen time, heighten our dependence on digital devices, and exacerbate issues such as digital distraction and information overload. Likewise, as virtual and augmented reality become more commonplace, we will need to navigate new boundaries between our digital and physical realities.

In this evolving landscape, staying informed and adaptable is essential. This means keeping abreast of the latest digital trends, understanding their potential impacts on our mental health, and adjusting our behaviors accordingly. It also involves continuing to prioritize our digital well-being, irrespective of the changes around us. This could mean maintaining our digital boundaries, practicing digital minimalism, and continuing to engage with technology in mindful, intentional ways.

Furthermore, we must remember the importance of critical thinking and digital literacy in this changing landscape. As technology becomes more sophisticated, our ability to assess online information, understand digital platforms, and make informed decisions about our digital behaviors will become increasingly important.

Finally, we must continue to advocate for a more resilient digital society. This involves fostering open communication about our digital experiences, promoting digital literacy and critical thinking, and working collaboratively to create digital environments that support, rather than undermine, our well-being.

While the future of the digital age is uncertain, what remains constant is our capacity for resilience, adaptation, and growth. As we navigate this evolving landscape, let's stay informed, adaptable, and intentional in our digital behaviors, ensuring that technology continues to serve us, rather than the other way around. The future of the digital age is ours to shape; let's make it one that supports our collective well-being.

Embracing the Digital Age Mindfully

Continuing the Journey of Digital Well-being

As we draw to the close of our exploration into digital well-being, it's essential to reflect on the journey we've undertaken together. In this digital age, it's clear that our interactions with technology can profoundly influence our mental health, relationships, productivity, and overall well-being. However, we also learned that we are not powerless in the face of these digital forces. Rather, we have the capacity to shape our digital experiences in ways that support our well-being.

We've discussed numerous strategies for cultivating digital resilience, from enhancing our digital literacy and critical thinking skills to practicing digital minimalism and detoxification. We've explored the importance of mindful technology use, the potential of online mental health resources, and the need for balance between our online and offline lives. And we've considered the future of the digital age and how we can stay informed and adaptable amidst its continual evolution.

Now, as we conclude this book, the challenge is to take these insights and apply them to our digital lives. We can use the strategies we've learned to navigate the digital world confidently and mindfully, making informed decisions about our digital behaviors, setting boundaries with technology, and using digital tools in ways that truly serve our needs.

Yet, as we have noted throughout, this isn't a one-size-fits-all endeavor. Each of us has unique digital needs, preferences, and challenges. Thus, it's crucial that we remain attuned to our individual experiences and continue to adapt our digital behaviors in ways that best support our well-being. There is no 'perfect' way to navigate the digital age, but by staying mindful, adaptable, and intentional, we can create digital lives that align with our values and support our mental health.

Moreover, let's remember that our journey of digital well-being doesn't end with this book. Instead, it's a continual process of learning, growing, and adapting. As technology evolves, new challenges and opportunities will undoubtedly arise, and we will need to adjust our strategies accordingly. Thus, it's essential to stay informed about the latest digital trends, continue to engage in critical thinking and self-reflection, and maintain open conversations about our digital experiences.

Let's embrace the digital age mindfully, intentionally, and confidently. Let's use the tools and strategies we've learned to navigate the digital world in ways that support our well-being. And let's continue our journey of digital well-being, staying adaptable and resilient in the face of the ever-evolving digital landscape. The future of the digital age is ours to shape, and with mindfulness and intentionality, we can make it one that supports our collective well-being.

About The Author

S. B. Sulzer has a rich background in global media, she isn't merely watching the impact of the digital aera unfold from the sidelines - she's been at the very heart of it.

Her journey has taken her across 20 countries through the US, Europe and the Middle-East, working with big-name entertainment companies, and leading their digital transformations. She's been at the core of the industry's inner workings, living and breathing audience engagement and content strategies. But her journey was about more than just business. It was about understanding the real power of media, the responsibilities that come with it, and the potential it holds - for better and for worse.

This book is her way of sharing her experiences and learnings. It's a blend of her professional insights, observations, and a desire to help shape a healthier relationship with our digital world. She's here to share knowledge, stimulate conversations, and inspire a positive change in our digital habits. This book is her story, told in a way that's easy to understand, relatable, and engaging for all ages. She invites you to join her on this enlightening journey towards a more balanced and healthier digital life.

www.sbsulzer.com

Bibliography

The Psychology of Screen Time
- Understanding Social Comparison on Social Media by The Jed Foundation
- Social comparison on social networking sites by Philippe Verduyn, Nino Gugushvili, Karlijn Massar, Karin Täht, Ethan Kross
- Digital Addiction and Sleep, Birgitta Dresp-Langley and Axel Hutt

The Dark Side of Constant Connectivity
- Associations between screen time and lower psychological well-being among children and adolescents: Evidence from a population-based study by Jean M. Twengea,* and W. Keith Campbellb, National Institutes of Health
- Digital Addiction and Compulsive Behavior
- Digital Addiction and Sleep, Birgitta Dresp-Langley and Axel Hutt

Gaming and Mental Health
- Exploring the Relationship Between Social Gaming, Anxiety and Loneliness by Deanna Herbert
- Is Increased Video Game Participation Associated With Reduced Sense of Loneliness? A Systematic Review and Meta-Analysis by Yan Luo,corresponding, Michelle Moosbrugger, Daniel M. Smith, Thaddeus J. France, Jieru Ma, and Jinxiang Xiao, National Institutes of Health
- Violent Video Games can Increase Aggression by Craig A. Anderson, Ph.D., and Karen E. Dill, Ph.D, American Psychological Association

- Violent Video Game Effects on Aggression, Empathy, and Prosocial Behavior in Eastern and Western Countries: A Meta-Analytic Review by Craig A. Anderson, Akiko Shibuya, Nobuko Ihori, Edward L. Swing, Brad J. Bushman, Akira Sakamoto, Hannah R. Rothstein, Muniba Saleem

Cyberbullying and Online Harassment
- A Majority of Teens Have Experienced Some Form of Cyberbullying, Pew Research Center
- Teens and Cyberbullying 2022, Pew Research Center